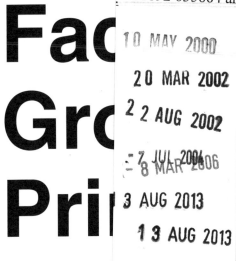

Fac
Gro
Prin

A manu

Marion

Tayside Centr
University of Dundee

RADCLIFFE MEDICAL PRESS

Radcliffe Medical Press
18 Marcham Road, Abingdon, Oxon OX14 1AA

ISBN 1 85775 401 8

Typeset by Joshua Associates Ltd, Oxford
Printed and bound by TJ International Ltd, Padstow, Cornwall

W 89
PRIMARY HC
TEAMWORK
GROUPS

Contents

Preface

In recent years general practice has provided an almost constant experience of change, much of it imposed.

Practices have been asked to become team based, to embrace new technology, to construct practice development plans, to devise multi-disciplinary protocols for managing patient care, to introduce regular audit procedures and now to present their 'practice perspective' to the Local Healthcare Co-operative or Primary Care Group.

There are many guides and manuals available, offering techniques for improving teamwork and for instigating and managing change – from *team development kits* to *SWOT analysis* to *needs assessment* to *action planning*. Few of these take a 'step back' to discuss **who** will guide the process and **what skills** those people will need.

This handbook draws on the experience of a number of research and development projects managed from The Tayside Centre for General Practice, University of Dundee, and is grounded in the work of modern day general practice in the United Kingdom. It does contain tips and techniques for improving the working of groups, but its central purpose is to equip those individuals working in general practice with an understanding of how people work together and how they can be helped to do that more effectively. With that aim in mind it will be of benefit to any member of the primary care team.

Facilitators are often used in business settings to assist groups with change. The role of the Facilitator is essentially to make something easier (*see* Chapter 3 for a more detailed description). Many practices have used *external* Facilitators in the past. While there may always be a place for them in some situations, we believe that individuals *in-house* can help to facilitate their own group, thus reducing the need for outside intervention.

Marion Duffy
Elaine Griffin
September 1999

List of tools

- Ice breakers
- Inlaws and outlaws
- Planning for a small group
- Clarifying the task and process of an existing group
- Reflections card game
- Root Cause Analysis
- Meetings Checklist
- Brainstorming
- A round
- Giving feedback

List of case studies

Acknowledgements

The authors gratefully acknowledge the financial support of Roche Pharmaceuticals without whose sponsorship this handbook, its sequel *Facilitating Organisational Change in Primary Care*, and the accompanying workshops, would not have been developed. Roche responded to a need, identified by the authors, for a handbook for those working in primary care that was contextualised for that setting. Facilitation posts are increasingly being advertised by healthcare organisations yet those who take on the task find little published material to help support their own development in the role. Additionally, practice-based professionals need to develop facilitation skills so that they can maximise the effectiveness of teamworking in the organisation and provision of healthcare.

Eight general medical practices from the Tayside and Grampian regions of Scotland participated in the workshops that accompanied the development of this handbook. Their active engagement in the skill development process and their feedback on the relevance and value of both the handbook and the training have been of considerable benefit to the authors. We extend our thanks to them.

Fifteen general medical practices in Tayside participated in the project entitled *Facilitating Education and Development* (The FED Project). Many of the case studies in this handbook are based on experiences during that project, although some details have been altered to ensure confidentiality. We acknowledge the practices' willing co-operation in that project.

We would also like to thank colleagues at Tayside Centre for General Practice and Tayside Audit Resource for Primary Care (TARPC) for sharing their past experiences of using facilitation as a tool for personal and practice development. In particular we mention Arlene Napier who gave generously of her time and resources in the development of the content for the handbook, and the Practice Audit Co-ordinator 'Sally' who gave an insight into facilitating audit in her own practice.

And finally, we must acknowledge the support and encouragement of our own families for whom the production of this handbook must have imprinted the name 'The Facpack' forever in their memories. Thank you for your encouragement and practical support.

Chapter 1

Introduction

Summary

The introduction describes the focus of the handbook as 'working in groups'.

It sets the context by helping you to focus on how your practice works together and describes a practice which used a Facilitator to help it establish its goals for development.

Please note that, for reasons of convenience, we refer throughout the handbook to the facilitator as of female gender. All references can be assumed to refer to facilitators of either gender.

This handbook looks at facilitating groups in primary care through knowledge and understanding of the context of general practice, and of how groups typically work together. As the need for meetings has increased in the current climate, the handbook focuses on what typically happens when groups work together in a meeting session and suggests an approach which uses facilitative behaviour to make that process of working together easier.

You will be asked to think about how *you* might act in a more facilitative way, and whether the formal role of *Facilitator* is one to which you might aspire.

Think now about your own practice:

• are your practice meetings productive?
• is everyone clear about their own and others' roles?
• are decisions always implemented?
• how do you handle conflicting views?
• do you discuss the potential effect any change might have?
• do you review your group's functioning from time to time?

Does anyone ask these questions about **your** practice? **Who** would answer them?

Here is a real life example from the Yellow Practice, a city centre practice with a team of 28 in total who dealt with some of the questions listed above. They called in an external Facilitator to help them move forward in developing their practice.

Case Study 1
Facilitating development
The Yellow Practice

The Yellow Practice was required to produce a Practice Development Plan by its local Health Board. The partners asked the Practice Manager to 'see to it' and she decided to get a group together comprising one representative from each of the main staff groups in the practice – GPs, practice nurses, district nurses, health visitors, reception staff and herself.

Twelve meetings took place over a six month period but attendance was patchy. The GP was usually 'too busy' to attend and there was always at least one member on holiday at any one time. However, the group had lots of ideas for developing the practice and spent many hours discussing them. Nevertheless, after six months there was still nothing in writing and the group was struggling to find a direction. The members of the group didn't know if all the practice members would like their plan and they were not sure whether they were supposed to be implementing as well as planning the development of the practice. Who would write the plan? Whose job was it really? Which decisions could they make and which ones would have to be referred back to the partners?

> The Health Board had sent round a reminder that plans should be submitted within the next six months. The Practice Manager asked a local Primary Care Facilitator to attend a practice development meeting and offer some advice. The Facilitator suggested that she would facilitate a meeting where the whole practice would get together to establish its goals for development (to include writing the development plan itself) based on a clear vision presented by the partners. They would then be in a position to devise a system whereby goals could be pursued in a way that had the commitment and support of the whole group. At that meeting the practice decided to form small working groups containing representatives from key staff groups to address a set of agreed goals. The Facilitator helped the first working group establish itself – and its way of working – and left some guidance which other groups could follow.

The critical help that the Facilitator gave was in helping the practice establish how it would achieve its own goals. She encouraged the practice team, through discussion, to be quite explicit about what was to be done, who would do it, what authority they would have and how the whole group would be kept informed.

Although the practice possessed lots of ideas and had set up a forum for discussing them, it had not devised a suitable mechanism whereby group ideas could be converted into **action** in a way that was designed by, and acceptable to, the whole practice.

The Facilitator's guidance came from her knowledge of how groups work and the particular context of general practice. Her skill was to run an effective meeting, help the group reach consensus on the next step, and offer some structure which would allow the small working groups to plan and reflect on their own operating procedures.

With training, guidance, experience and reflection, **you**, or someone in your practice, can develop facilitation skills which might help your practice in similar ways. These skills can also be transferred to other settings where you are part of a group – perhaps you run a carers' group or are a member of a local committee, or participate in a professional working group.

Chapter 2

How to use this handbook

Summary

This chapter gives a guide to the content and structure of the handbook, explaining the role of:

- *theory*
- *reference to general practice*
- *case studies from local projects*
- *suggestions for facilitating your own practice*
- *tips and tools to help you facilitate.*

The handbook is divided into three main sections:

1 A general introduction to facilitation skills
2 How groups work
3 Making meetings more effective.

There is also a summary chapter entitled *Qualities, skills and opportunities.* You may want to read this chapter first to gain an overview of the content of the handbook.

In each of the three main sections you will find:

Theory A brief overview of some of the relevant body of knowledge.

General Practice	How theory translates to real life in general practice.
Case Study	An example from general practice.
Tips and Tools	For diagnosing difficulties, suggesting alternative ways of working and encouraging a more reflective approach to working together – all tried and tested in the context of general practice.
Facilitate Your Own Practice	How **you** can help smooth the process of managing in this climate of change in general practice.

For easy access descriptions of specific facilitation tools and techniques referred to in the text, are marked with the symbol:

Other aids to facilitation appear in the body of the chapter and are surrounded by a border like this:

Chapter 3

A general introduction to facilitation skills

Summary

In this chapter, we develop your understanding of the skills and personal qualities required of a Facilitator.

Reference is made to several key writers on facilitation who help us describe the role of the Facilitator – John Heron, Trevor Bentley and Dale Hunter and colleagues.

We relate facilitation to six aspects of the functioning of a group and point to the need for flexibility in leadership style.

We highlight some of the work done by facilitators in the Health Service over the last 15 years, particularly in relation to developing practice teams. The supply and effectiveness of external Facilitators is discussed and contrasted with those of internal Practice Audit Co-ordinators.

We invite you to consider your own suitability to act in a Facilitator role in your own practice or group, outlining some key behaviours that a Facilitator must employ and others that should be avoided. John Heron's 'criteria for excellence' in the role of facilitating the development of others' interpersonal skills are also detailed.

> ### Theory

What is facilitation?

As the dictionary defines, to 'facilitate' is to 'make something easier'. Facilitators ease a group through the process of making a decision, solving a problem, redefining goals, or introducing change – helping others make a movement by guiding the process.

According to Bentley (1994) the Facilitator will:

- provide opportunities for the group to go in the direction they want to go
- be constantly aware of what is happening in the group
- stay quiet, and attentive, to the needs of individuals in the group.

The work of John Heron (1989) has guided many Facilitators. He described the role of the Facilitator as being one which considers six aspects of the functioning of the group:

1 *planning*: how will the group acquire its objectives and establish a programme?
2 *meaning*: how will members of the group make sense of what is going on?
3 *confronting*: how will the group become conscious of its own resistance to facing and dealing with certain issues?
4 *feeling*: how will the emotional life of the group be handled?
5 *structuring*: how will the group actively work together?
6 *valuing*: how can a climate of personal value, integrity and respect be created?

The Facilitator can choose at any point to either:

- direct the group, do things for it and lead from the front (*the hierarchical mode*)
- share power and manage *with* the group (*the co-operative mode*)
- give the group freedom to find its own way without reminders, guidance or assistance (*the autonomous mode*).

Key to effective facilitation is being able to operate in a **flexible** way to meet the needs of the group at any one point.

Bentley (1994) encapsulated the work of the Facilitator concisely in this description:

'Facilitation is the provision of opportunity, resources, encouragement and support for the group to succeed in achieving its own objectives and to do this through enabling the group to take control and responsibility for the way they proceed.'

It is clear that facilitation skills are needed in modern group practice to meet the challenges of shared care, team-based planning, health needs assessment and so on. Now read on to find out how facilitation in primary care has been employed in recent times.

General Practice

Facilitators in the NHS

As a development process, facilitation has been part of the business world for many years now. During the last 15 years it has also been used increasingly in primary healthcare. In the late 1990s, there are in excess of 500 people working as Facilitators in the National Health Service, and at least 160 are entitled 'Primary Care Facilitators'. Support for these Facilitators is available from the National Primary Care Facilitation Project, based in Oxford.*

In the past, facilitators have worked successfully with general practices to:

- organise study days on clinical topics such as diabetes
- implement and manage an immunisation programme
- support practice nurses in asthma audit
- improve detection and management of cardiovascular risk factors
- improve early detection of cancer
- increase acceptance of a breast screening service by ethnic minority groups
- involve large numbers of GPs in the shared care of drug users
- run or manage away days
- help with the production of practice development plans
- assist with patient satisfaction surveys and analysis
- help with information management and technology.

(The National Primary Care Facilitation Programme, 1998)

In contrast to Case Study 1, here is an example of where an *internal member of staff* worked closely on a one-to-one basis with an *external* Facilitator to develop her own in-house audit facilitation skills.

---

* The National Primary Care Facilitation Programme, Block 10, The Churchill, Headington, Oxford OX3 7LJ.

Case Study 2
Facilitating audit
Sally

The Green Practice was invited by its Regional Audit Manager to nominate a member of staff to become a Practice Audit Co-ordinator. She would receive training and support in planning, implementing and managing audit projects in the practice and the intention was that the practice would eventually integrate audit into its regular activity. Sally was offered the post and given additional hours each week to enable her to develop the necessary skills to put audit into practice. It was a bonus that she already had well-developed computer skills, having used the GPASS medical records software on a daily basis in her role as Computer Operator in the practice.

A Health Board Audit Facilitator (Claire) worked with Sally and staff from other local practices. In their first year Claire ran workshops in *Introduction to clinical audit*, *Report writing skills for audit*, *Questionnaire design*, *Presentation skills*, *Audit quality and guidelines*. She helped the Practice Audit Co-ordinators develop computer skills in word processing, database, spreadsheet and electronic presentation. She supported their efforts back in their practices and was available for specific practical help such as analysing data or compiling an audit report. Just as important, she also offered immediate, accessible, individual moral support and advice. Sally felt she could approach the Facilitator at any time, however insignificant her problem or need might appear.

After a year, Sally had developed practical skills in collecting and analysing data. She formally presented audit information, about management of patients with diabetes within the practice, to the rest of the practice and produced a report on the audit work. She liaised with the 'audit' GP in the practice as necessary and with confidence. She summed up the experience in this way:

> '*The training has allayed many of my fears about undertaking audit. I felt some pride in completing a piece of work, presenting it to the practice and providing a tool for moving the practice on in its care of diabetic patients. Now I would like to develop some more facilitation skills which will equip me to manage feedback meetings, help the practice come to decisions and implement changes to really take things forward.*'

Many of these skills will be developed through a Facilitation Skills Training Programme in year two of Sally's Practice Audit Co-ordinator course.

The Health Board Audit Facilitator in this case study worked as director, guide and support to the Practice Audit Co-ordinators in the process of developing their audit, interpersonal and communication skills. Sally's view was that the help of the Facilitator had been the key to her progress so far. This facilitation model has been used effectively to integrate audit into practice life in more than 40 Tayside practices (Grant *et al.*, 1998). Its ultimate success will be measured by the extent to which the Practice Audit Co-ordinators can fully facilitate and co-ordinate audit projects within their own practices.

Facilitators and the development of practice teams

Facilitators have been used perhaps most effectively in the development of practice teams. Havelock (1997) points to the different types of help that practices need, based on the particular stage of development and sophistication evident in the practice team.

Basic level: the Facilitator can help with the production of the practice development plan or can encourage the professional development of practice staff.

Level Two: he/she can support multi-disciplinary workshops and study days which allow the team to learn together and develop plans, e.g. for chronic disease management.

Level Three: once the team has started to work together more, the Facilitator can help to develop more effective meetings or arrange strategic planning away days.

Level Four: with an increased sense of teamwork the Facilitator can encourage and support health needs assessment, local community group involvement in healthcare, or a Total Quality Management Programme within the practice.

Limitations to using external facilitators

However useful external Facilitators are, there are limitations to their role and effectiveness. 'The Facilitator Effect' described by McCowan *et al.* (1997) demonstrates how the practice can revert to its original way of working once the Facilitator has left the practice. Furthermore, Facilitators with an in-depth knowledge and understanding of the context of primary care are not always easy to find, and those without that knowledge may be perceived as less credible by practice members. Additionally, it may be a problem finding funds to pay for these services.

Hooker (1994) summed up the situation well when he said:

> 'In the UK the process of change in primary care seems unlikely to abate. The need for a continued facilitation presence appears assured, but what form it will take is less sure. Although there will clearly be a need in the UK for the specialist role of facilitating primary healthcare to continue, I would propose . . . as managers are learning from the success of facilitation in achieving change, they could increasingly adopt a more facilitatory style.'

We suggest that not only managers, but **all members** of the primary healthcare team adopt a more facilitatory style.

How would you start to develop a more facilitatory style? How would it need to differ from your normal style? You may find it difficult to answer these questions but this handbook is designed to help you do so.

As you read through this handbook you will consider the desirable qualities, skills and attitudes exhibited by a Facilitator – from the standpoint of both the recognised experts and from local experience of the use of external Facilitators in general practice. We will then build on that knowledge to help you develop **your** facilitative skills.

Facilitate Your Own Practice

How *you* can act in a facilitative way

There are two main ways in which you can facilitate your own practice – first, by acting as Facilitator for particular activities or events (e.g. away days), and second, by behaving in a way that helps your particular group reach decisions, handle conflict and maximise its potential (whether it be, for example, an integrated nursing team, a practice management group, a prescribing guidelines working party or full primary healthcare team). In the second book in this series, *Facilitating Organisational Change in Primary Care*, information is given on running away days and planning an organisational development programme – the *practical* aspects of facilitating the process so that the job is done well. Developing skills to facilitate the interaction between members of a group, however, comes less from following a checklist and more from understanding yourself, the group and your relationship with it. We expand on this aspect of facilitation later on in this handbook.

Are you suited to the formal Facilitator role?

In considering how suited you might be to the formal Facilitator role you might want to consider the following questions posed by Dale Hunter *et al.* (1996):

* do I want to dominate this group?
* do I feel dominated by this group?
* am I afraid of this group?
* do I know what is best for this group?
* do I like/agree with some members of this group and not others?
* am I the only person who will work well with this group?

If the answer to any of these is 'Yes', you may need to think again about how suited you are to this role. Remember our earlier definition of facilitation?

> '. . . the provision of opportunity, resources, encouragement and support for the group to succeed in achieving its own objectives and to do this through enabling the group to take control and responsibility for the way they proceed.'

To fulfil this role is to leave the 'I' behind – my needs, wants, problems, relationship difficulties, personal agenda – to work instead for the benefit of the group. It takes a certain courage and requires sufficient self-awareness to admit your possible shortcomings in the role and, above all, a willingness to 'go with the flow' of the group.

Tips and Tools

Taking on the formal Facilitator role may entail quite a different set of behaviours from those you normally display in a group. Reflect on the key principles of facilitating a group – and think about how many of these tasks you would normally attend to when you work with colleagues in groups.

Key principles of facilitating a group

In order to facilitate a group the Facilitator has to:

- listen attentively and actively to participants
- deal with interruptions and conflict
- be aware of the energy of the group and how to sustain it
- support the group
- be fully engaged with the group
- protect freedom of expression and activity
- invite participation
- release the potential of the group.

We expand on these ideas later.

Types of behaviour for the Facilitator to avoid

It will help your understanding to recognise that there are some types of behaviour which the Facilitator would do well to *avoid* employing:

- working to her own hidden agenda
- controlling the group process without attention to what the group wants
- persuading the group to accept her ideas, and not theirs
- choosing not to recognise what is really happening in the group
- using power and authority to feed her own ego
- rescuing people rather than supporting and encouraging them.

Varying your leadership style

The Facilitator role may sometimes mean leading from the front, giving direction, providing a structure, bringing resources, planning activities – but it is how you do that which is important. For example, if there are planned objectives and timescales and procedures, declare what they are and allow room for change by the group – avoid making decisions without the group's involvement. It may also entail acting as expert on occasions – but that is done with the agreement of, or at the request of, the group inviting your expert contribution for a specific purpose.

The relationship between the Facilitator and the group

Understanding how groups work is considered in Chapter 4, but as a starting point to understanding the Facilitator role, the following is instructive.

- The role of Facilitator to a group is quite different to that of manager or group leader where most of the control and accountability rests with the manager/leader. The Facilitator role is given by the group, to whom the Facilitator is then responsible and accountable. It recognises the importance of the process of the group and the need for it to have a guide.
- It is important for the group and the Facilitator to be quite clear what the Facilitator role entails.
- A group is more than the sum of its parts and may be capable of much more than each individual thinks is possible. This is known as *synergy*. The Facilitator is out to tap the energy of the group and so stimulate synergy.

(Hunter *et al.*, 1996)

Criteria for excellence in the Facilitator role

Heron's (1989) own criteria for excellence in the role of facilitating the development of interpersonal skills within a group include the following:

- you can confront supportively
- you can provide orientation in the course of work
- you come over as caring, warm and genuine
- you have a wide repertoire of techniques for personal and interpersonal development
- you can fully respect the autonomy of the other person
- you can show flexibility of style.

It may be that the formal Facilitator role does not attract you, or perhaps you can already see aspects of the role which would be alien to you. As we have already suggested, however, all of us can begin to act in a generally more facilitative way. We develop this aspect further in Chapter 4, identifying *how* and *where*, and beginning with a look at how groups tend to work.

Chapter 4

How groups work

Summary

We begin this chapter by describing:

- *the advantages of working in groups*
- *the stages in the evolution of a group*
- *the milestones to 'synergy'*
- *the indicators of an effective group*
- *the conditions which impair the workings of a group*
- *the teams and groups in general practice*
- *the problems which typically occur in primary healthcare teams.*

We point to where you can have a facilitative effect in:

- *setting up a new group*
- *improving the functioning of an existing group*
- *behaving in a more effective way as a group member.*

We highlight behaviour which:

- *helps, hinders or even destroys groups*
- *gets the job done*
- *helps group members to work together more harmoniously.*

We then describe some tools to:

- *clarify the task and process of an existing group*
- *set up a new group.*

And some tips on how to:

- *employ good listening and speaking skills*
- *facilitate groups generally*
- *intervene in an appropriate way in particular situations.*

Theory

The advantages of working in groups

In a world of increasing complexity it is common practice to use groups to generate ideas, make decisions and solve problems. The theoretical advantages to using groups are typically identified as:

- several people make more 'man hours' available
- information and skills can be pooled
- more ideas are likely to be generated
- a greater *variety* of ideas is generated
- errors are more likely to be spotted
- increased involvement equals increased commitment.

In reality, these theoretical advantages are often counteracted by the kinds of operational difficulties that occur when a group evolves through a number of stages. Heron (1989) described these stages as 'wintertime, springtime, summertime and autumn'. Others have used the terms 'forming, storming, norming, performing' or 'orientation, dissatisfaction, resolution, production and termination'. Whatever the exact terminology, the underlying concept is that the group undergoes a shift in functioning from negative to positive forms.

The stages in the evolution of a group

The process has been described as a cyclical one:

- *wintertime*: where the ground is frozen and the weather stormy – trust within the group is low and anxiety is high

- *springtime*: where new life starts to break through. Trust is building, anxiety is reducing. If conditions are suitable, a new culture is created
- *summertime*: where there is an abundance of growth and the sun is high. Here there is openness, risk taking, working, caring and sharing
- *autumn*: when the fruit is harvested and stored. The group draws to a close, members review the fruit of their work and there may be some distress at parting.

(Heron, 1989)

Unaided, not all groups move successfully to 'summertime'. The role of the Facilitator can be to help the group move from the negative to more positive forms, and so more fully realise the benefits of working in a group. The Facilitator will recognise the typical patterns exhibited by groups at different stages in their life cycle.

Some typical characteristics of the *undeveloped group* or team are that: the undeveloped group tends not to deal with feelings; members conform rather than rock the boat; there may be no shared understanding of what has to be done; mistakes are covered up by individuals for fear of indicating failure; people confine themselves to their own defined jobs; and the boss takes most of the decisions (Woodcock, 1989).

In contrast, the *experimenting team* is willing to experiment, review its operations, face problems and consider a range of options before making decisions. There is more listening at meetings and less talking. Feelings begin to be considered.

The *consolidating team* adopts a more systematic approach to its task, agreeing rules and procedures and making decisions in a structured way. Improved relationships are maintained and used productively.

A mature team is flexible, recognises which type of leadership is required, is committed to its own development and is a happy, rewarding place to be.

As Hunter *et al.* (1996) remind us:

'a purposeful group is not just a collection of individuals. A group is an entity in itself. It is a living system with its own physical form, its own personality, its own potential and its own limitations.'

As with all living systems it will flourish if the conditions are right, and facilitation can help the group move through Hunter's milestones to synergy – a pathway to working together harmoniously and productively.

Milestones to synergy

- The group has a clear purpose and group members are committed to it.
- The group develops a powerful vision which continues to inspire members when the going gets tough.
- Values are discussed and referred to when making tough decisions.
- The group clarifies roles and commitments, e.g. expectations and limits.
- The group designs and implements projects to achieve its purpose.
- Group members develop a group identity. Group members share honestly with each other and so develop trust.
- Conflict is seen as normal and is worked through rather than avoided.
- Group members acknowledge contributions to the group and celebrate accomplishments.

If you have experienced true synergy you will know that it is more than the sum of the milestones listed above. It can be exciting, lively, satisfying, rewarding and immensely reassuring. Even if your group is not truly synergistic in its operations, how do you know when a group is working effectively? Indicators of an effective group might include the following.

Indicators of an effective group

- A relaxed and comfortable environment where group members are involved and interested.
- Widespread and regular participation in discussion which is relevant to the task in hand.
- Active listening by all with every idea given a hearing.
- Most decisions reached by genuine consensus rather than by voting or by withholding disagreement.
- Constructive criticism in order to remove obstacles to progress.
- Clear action plans made.
- Leadership according to circumstances and need and not status or convention.
- A reflective element in the group operation to review its own procedures or activities.

Conditions which impair the workings of a group

We look now in detail at some of the conditions which typically *impair* the working of a group in order to begin to see where a Facilitator can be of help.

Using Heron's classification, these can be described as:

- overconcentration on one type of activity, e.g. intellectual activity
- competitiveness
- control and suppression of feelings
- habitual inequality in contribution to the group
- power struggles
- gender bias
- compulsive focus on the task
- emotional and physical isolation
- anxiety about being part of the group and also anxiety present in individuals from their past experience of life.

(Heron, 1989)

Going into these aspects in more detail:

Overconcentration on one aspect of the group can happen in a number of different ways and with different consequences. When members interact only on an intellectual basis their interactions may be emotionally dead, with no sharing of personal experience. They relate to each other in a closed, restricted and detached kind of way. Alternatively, when the group focuses too heavily on personal and interpersonal development the reverse kind of alienation can occur, where members become immersed in sharing emotional experiences and pay scant attention to the intellectual aspect.

Heron described other forms of alienation – of the spirit and from the body. The basic tenet is that groups function best when they integrate body, mind and spirit.

Competitiveness can be endemic in the culture – the group may foster the value of competition for status, competence and power.

Control and suppression of feelings may become accepted behaviour so that there is limited expression of positive feelings and total suppression of distress feelings. Both of these restrict behaviour in the group.

Social restrictions to effective group functioning include:

- **habitual inequality** in contributions to the group, where some members habitually dominate discussion and others say little or nothing
- **power struggles** where high contributors try to railroad their decisions through
- **gender bias** where men speak and act first and women's perspectives or initiatives are suppressed (the reverse is rare!)
- **compulsive focus on the task** where there is pressure to fill all working time with some clearly defined or familiar kind of task
- **emotional and physical isolation** where people keep themselves emotionally buttoned-up and physically apart.

The **anxieties** of participants also inhibit full and effective participation in the group. These anxieties can arise from being in the group – about being accepted, liked and wanted; about understanding what is going on and being understood by others; about being competent and exercising sufficient control over events to meet one's own needs. Heron (1989) also described 'archaic anxiety' which represents distress felt in earlier experiences, particularly childhood ones – the distress of being rejected or being overwhelmed by external events for example. The anxiety of being in the group can stir up pain which has not been adequately dealt with in the past. Most people will carry around at least some of this so-called 'baggage'.

Mindful of the potential for certain conditions to impair the functioning of the group, the Facilitator's job is to make it easier for the group to achieve its purpose and to empower the group to tap into its synergistic potential. How to do this comes later. First, we look at how general practice groups tend to work.

General Practice

Teams and groups in general practice

In everyday conversation in general practice, the word 'team' is often used to describe the groups which work together to provide practice-based primary care. A 'team' is essentially a group of people organised to work together and in any medical practice a 'team' of people will engage in:

- the diagnosis, treatment and management of acute and chronic conditions
- antenatal and postnatal care, and access to contraceptive advice and provision
- prevention of disease and disability

- the follow-up and continuing care of chronic and recurring disease
- rehabilitation after illness
- care during terminal illness
- the co-ordination of services for those at risk, including children, the mentally ill, the bereaved, the elderly, the handicapped and those who care for them
- helping patients and their relatives to make appropriate use of other agencies for care and support including hospital-based specialists.

(RCGP, 1998)

The exact composition of any primary healthcare team will depend on factors such as the overall aims of the team and the needs of the practice population. Different groups within the team will come together at different times to enable the whole caring process to take place – for example, the practice management group, the practice nursing team, the community nursing team, the clinical team, the practice development group, the prescribing guidelines group. In all of these the *theory* is that, as before:

- several people make more 'man hours' available
- information and skills are pooled
- more ideas are likely to be generated
- a greater variety of ideas is generated
- errors are more likely to be spotted
- increased involvement equals increased commitment

and that *synergy* – the potential within the group – is released.

What tends to happen in reality is more like the following case study from a six doctor rural practice, with a 21 member primary healthcare team, who were attempting to work as a team to produce a practice development plan.

Case Study 3
Task focused group
The Red Practice

The Red Practice was a busy practice situated in a rural area in the West of Scotland, much frequented by tourists. The senior partner belonged to 'the old school' and believed that doctors should care for their own individual lists of patients and do everything possible to help them, regardless of the hour or the nature of the demand. He tended to make most of the major decisions in the practice although he believed that he did consult with colleagues but found them strangely apathetic or not robust enough to cope with the challenges of general practice.

The Practice Manager was trying to introduce a more team-based approach to planning, support and delivery of care but was hampered by a number of factors including the location of the community nurses who were based in another health centre. The practice staff by and large also attended the practice as patients and found it difficult to separate their professional and personal relationships with the doctors. Working together on the production of a practice development plan might have provided the vehicle for developing the primary healthcare team.

A working group was appointed comprising a representative from each of the staff groups in the practice, i.e. one GP, one practice nurse, one community nurse and so on. That representative consulted with his/her colleagues to find out their views on the future of the practice, e.g. the Practice Nurse on the working group would liaise with her practice nurse colleagues. These representatives put together a draft list of practice goals based on the views of their respective colleagues and finally the whole primary care team got together to discuss the list, with the senior partner leading the discussion.

At that meeting a number of things happened. Some members of staff never once lifted their eyes from the floor, others shifted in their seats and exhibited signs of discomfort; there was considerable unspoken resistance to ideas; the senior partner tended to dominate the discussion; some of the reception staff said nothing at all; team members were reticent about agreeing or disagreeing with any proposals; the air was heavy with silence on occasions. The senior partner struggled to keep momentum going and achieve any consensus. At the end of the meeting a list of goals *was* established but there was no air of synergy, no sense of satisfaction with a job well done. The word later was that the meeting had done nothing to improve teamworking.

What was going on in that group?

There are many examples here of behaviour which give clues to underlying problems in the group. Feelings were not dealt with; there was considerable anxiety about participating; some members brought 'baggage' from previous encounters; team members' willingness to contribute ideas or comments was affected by their position in the 'hierarchy'; there was no commitment to work for the benefit of the group; conflict was neither openly expressed nor dealt with. To a certain extent there was even increased rejection of the idea of becoming a team. Above all, there was no discussion on how the group was working, no focus on the process as opposed to the task.

If not as extreme, many primary healthcare teams or groups show similar problems in working together effectively.

Problems which typically occur in primary healthcare teams

- There may be status differences within the team which inhibit participation, where more junior or non-clinical staff feel reticent about speaking up.
- The practice may adhere to traditional patterns of authority and communication where information is not freely shared nor all staff consulted.
- Some staff groups may rarely come into contact with each other due to geographical distance or lack of opportunities to meet.
- Roles within groups tend not to be made explicit – for example, who will lead the group, who will organise the practicalities of meetings, whose job is it to check if decisions made are implemented?
- Pressures of time mean that there is a focus on achieving the end result, e.g. making a decision on a new telephone system, at the expense of maintaining effective working relationships.
- There may be some resistance to change, particularly in the wake of many years of imposed change, which affects enthusiasm and commitment within a group.
- There may be professional rivalry or antagonism such that working relationships are neither relaxed nor co-operative.
- Some groups may show signs of 'groupthink', where the group becomes isolated from outside influence and tends not to be critical of its own actions and decisions, reaching consensus too quickly and without proper debate.
- Time spent working in groups may seem wasted and unproductive with lots of talk and little action.
- Some members of the group have skills, experience, ideas and potentially valuable contributions that are not adequately recognised or used.

Practice teams don't often consider it necessary to look at how the team operates, and which values or principles should underpin decision making. Nor do they discuss and agree its exact purpose, clarify individuals' responsibilities to the team, or establish how it will review its own progress. Hardly surprising then if they fail to reach many of Hunter *et al.*'s 'Milestones to synergy' (*see* p. 20).

Armed with a better understanding of how groups work, and of the typical features of groups in primary care, how can you help as an individual to facilitate groups within your practice?

Facilitate Your Own Practice

There may be three areas in which you can have a facilitative effect.

1   When a new group is being set up you can suggest that it actively works to develop into an effective team. You can give some indication and guidance on how that might be done, facilitating the process yourself if that is appropriate within your group. There will be some specific tools for that described later in this section.
2   In an existing group, particularly if there is a feeling that it is not as productive as it might be, you could suggest some activities which would help improve the functioning of the group and offer to facilitate the group in those activities. Again, some examples of such activities are included in this section.
3   As a group member you can begin to behave in a generally more effective way, employing some quite specific types of intervention geared towards improving the interaction between group members.

Looking at the third option first – how should effective group members behave?

Helping and hindering behaviour in groups

You may want to follow the example of Hart (1992) where *helping* and *hindering roles* and *behaviours* found in groups are described. These behaviours help or hinder the group in working together in a co-operative and productive process to achieve its objectives.

Some roles or behaviours focus more on the task in hand, others on the working relationships and interpersonal issues which underpin the task. The latter concern, for example, morale, atmosphere, influence, participation, conflict, co-operation. Behaviour which hinders tends to serve the needs of the individual rather than the group. In thinking how you might help the group *get the job done* there are a number of roles you might adopt or behaviour you can choose to exhibit.

Roles and behaviours that help to get the job done: related to the task and the timescale

- **Initiating**

  Proposing tasks or goals; suggesting ways of getting the job done; identifying where problems lie

- **Information or opinion seeking**

  Asking for information from others; asking for ideas, suggestions, opinions

- **Information or opinion giving**

  Providing relevant information to the group; stating your own opinions; giving ideas and suggestions

- **Clarifying**

  Interpreting ideas of others; giving examples to elucidate suggestions; pointing out alternatives; defining terms

- **Summarising**

  Pulling together related ideas; restating what has been discussed; offering a decision or conclusion to be accepted or rejected by the group

- **Checking consensus**

  Checking to see how much agreement there is within the group and how ready the group is to make a decision

The skill of the effective group member is in using these types of behaviour at the *appropriate times*. Other helpful behaviours more concerned with the *process* of working together in a group are described in the following box.

Roles and behaviours that help the group to work well together: continuous and related to the process

• **Encouraging**	Being friendly, warm and responsive to others; giving others an opportunity to contribute or be recognised; accepting others and what they have to contribute
• **Harmonising**	Reducing tension; helping others to express their feelings; trying to reconcile disagreements
• **Expressing group feelings**	Sensing the mood of the group, the feelings and relationships within it; sharing your own feelings with the group
• **Gatekeeping**	Helping to keep communication channels open; suggesting procedures that encourage participation
• **Compromising**	Admitting your own mistakes; modifying your ideas in the interest of the group; offering a compromise even where it involves some loss of status
• **Standard setting and testing**	Checking whether the group is satisfied with its own procedures; suggesting new procedures if necessary; monitoring that the group is maintaining standards

You may be familiar with certain individual roles which hinder or destroy the group – you may have witnessed these in action. Have you also been guilty of such behaviour on occasions?

Roles that meet individual rather than group needs

- **The blocker** — who tends to reject ideas out of hand without considering them and may use status as a way of doing that
- **The critic** — who works for status in the group by criticising others and deflating their egos
- **The dominator** — who asserts authority or superiority to manipulate the group; who interrupts others and may adopt a patronising tone
- **The saboteur** — who disrupts the work of others and fools around
- **The withdrawer** — who acts passively, shows indifference, answers only briefly
- **The avoider** — who changes the topic or is frequently absent
- **The sympathy seeker** — who always brings the conversation back to his/her own personal concerns and problems
- **The sycophant** — who curries favour with the group leader

We suggest that if you try actively to tailor your own behaviour to the needs of the group you will be a more effective and facilitative group member.

Facilitating improvement in an existing group

In an existing group, members may be well aware that they are not working together productively or harmoniously. Your role as a member of that group with an interest in facilitating some improvement could be to suggest that the group takes time out to look at its working processes and culture, with the aim of improving the quality of the teamworking. Most members would probably benefit from a greater understanding of how groups work and it may be that you can create an opportunity to impart some of your knowledge to them in a general way without direct reference to your particular group.

You might want to flag up key aspects of groupworking such as:

- the benefits of working in groups
- the stages of group life
- the signposts to synergy

- the task and process elements
- the need to attend to the life of the group and not just the job to be done
- where groups typically have problems.

Clarifying the task and process of an existing group

You might then suggest that the group work together through a number of questions that encourage discussion and clarification in order to define the task and process of the group.

A full description of how to use the tool appears at the end of this chapter (*see* p. 47). Meanwhile, here are the questions the group would discuss.

Goals
- Are we all here for a common purpose?
- What is our task in this group?
- Do we need to revise our goals?
- How will we know when we have completed our task?

Roles
- Is the composition of the group appropriate?
- Who does what in this group?
- Is everyone clear about their own role?
- Is everyone clear about others' roles?
- Are we each able to fulfil our role?
- Can any constraints to carrying out our roles be reduced?

Procedures
- Do we meet often enough to achieve our aims?
- Do we waste time?
- Do we make it easy for everyone to contribute their ideas and opinions or do we let one or two do all the talking?
- Does everyone feel comfortable about challenging statements made in the group?
- Do we handle conflict effectively in the group?
- Do we make sure we have all the appropriate information available before making decisions?
- Do we specify who will implement any decisions?
- Do we follow up decisions and review the outcome?

Relationships
- How is morale within the group?
- Are we sensitive to how other people are feeling?
- Can we tolerate failure and give support rather than blame?

To create and sustain a climate where individuals will discuss these types of questions openly and constructively requires certain facilitative skills. We discuss these in **Tips and Tools**.

Facilitating a new group

Much of what you have already read in this chapter will be relevant if you are facilitating a new group. However, it is important to make the distinction between being a group member and being a group Facilitator. If you are simply a member of the group acting in your customary role of Practice Nurse or GP, then you can make use of facilitative behaviour and the techniques described above.

If you are a regular member of a new group you might find it useful to suggest that the group follows a format which proved useful when a prescribing group was being set up in a local city practice, where members of the group were keen to be as productive as possible.

Case Study 4
Setting up a new group
The Violet Practice

Prescribing Group: First Meeting, 30 May 1999

Discussion points for first meeting

- What is the role of this group? (remit, authority)
- What do we think we ought to be doing? (objectives)
- When and where are we going to meet? (venue and timetable suitable to participants which will allow us to complete the task)
- How are we going to work together in the group? (procedures, decision-making techniques)
- Do we need a group leader/co-ordinator? (alternative ways of working)
- What do we want to avoid doing?
- Do we want to have any ground rules for the way we operate? (attendance, commitment, helpful behaviour, dealing with conflicting views)
- What are the reporting arrangements? (do we need minutes, who will do them, what will be in them, who gets them?)

Taking on the formal Facilitator role

If you are to take on the formal role of Facilitator, however, it is important to clarify for yourself and the group how this will work.

As the Facilitator, you will be guiding the process and will not really be involved in the content of the group sessions. It probably would not work to pop in and out of the Facilitator role, trying to take part in decision making as well as facilitating. The group may make decisions with which you do not agree. Can you accept that?

You will also need to ascertain whether all members of the group can accept you as the Facilitator. That may be difficult if you normally express strong views or are seen to be associated with one particular faction within the group. Perhaps a colleague can monitor your neutrality and give you feedback at the end of a group session. It may also work for your group if the role of Facilitator is rotated amongst several within the group who have the necessary skills. This then allows you to play your normal role on occasions.

How can you use those types of skills and display some of those qualities in order to be more facilitative?

Tips and Tools

The two primary skills of facilitating

In common with other writers on facilitation skills Hunter *et al.* (1996) point to the two primary skills of facilitation: listening and speaking.

Listening is a very important part of facilitation. For most people, listening is full of assessments and judgements about the person who is speaking. It may also be a time when you rehearse what you are going to say next. In facilitation, however, your listening should be active and focused, and should communicate that you understand and value the person speaking. You have to listen for what the *individual* is saying not only in words but also in body language, tone of voice, expression – drawing forth the essence of what the other is thinking. On another level you listen for the mood, the purpose, the energy and the direction of the *group*. It is very hard work!

Speaking in a facilitative way is like using your voice as a musical instrument to support, initiate, clarify, encourage, calm, inspire, motivate and direct. What you say as a Facilitator is also known as *intervention*. It has a specific purpose for the benefit of the group, be it to encourage co-operation, break down barriers to progress, or lighten the atmosphere. You cannot plan the actual interventions in advance – they are dependent on what needs to be spoken for the benefit of the group. However, you can become familiar with a range of interventions which will give you a feel for how a Facilitator works. The Practice Audit Co-ordinators mentioned earlier, when facilitating meetings to review the progress of audit projects, were advised in the TARPC Facilitation Skills Training Course to do the following when facilitating a practice feedback meeting on their audit projects:

- remain neutral
- keep the focus
- be positive
- encourage participation
- protect ideas
- avoid evaluating
- suggest groupworking methods such as brainstorming
- share observations with the group
- co-ordinate practical details – setting out the room, organising any printed information etc.

(TARPC, 1999)

Some general guidelines for a group Facilitator acting to guide the process of the groupwork are given in the following box (after Hunter *et al.*, 1996).

General guidelines for facilitating groups

- Remember that a group is capable of more than any one member thinks is possible. By tapping the energy of the group you can create synergy.
- Trust that the group has the resources to achieve its task and work through the process. Display that confidence and encourage full exploration of the group's resources – ideas, knowledge, skills, strengths, enthusiasm, commitment etc.
- Always treat each member as if he/she is capable, fully functioning and committed to the purpose of the group even if their behaviour seems to show otherwise.
- Ensure that the physical environment is protected from interruptions and distractions.
- Always bear in mind the purpose of the group. Remind others of it if the group gets bogged down or diverted.
- Be adaptable and respond to what is going on at that moment. You cannot completely plan ahead.

Cont

- Remember that beginnings are crucial – getting started in a new group is like laying the foundations of the house. You need to make time to do this properly.
- Take everything that happens in the group as relevant, so that even 'falling off a chair' is part of the group process.
- Work with conflict, encourage others to express it openly and try to reach a resolution.
- Be 100% attentive at all times to what is going on in the group.
- Allow your own personality to shine through. You do not need to be stiff and formal – in fact, that may lead the group to behave in the same way.
- Do not judge others but do discern what is going on and intervene if appropriate. When are people 'switching off'? Are they aware of it? Are others frustrated? Discern when these and other non-productive types of behaviour are present and intervene as necessary.
- Don't take personally, and be tempted to comment on, ideas or beliefs expressed in the group, nor any criticism even if directed forcibly at yourself. If it happens keep a note of the 'trigger' and learn from the experience.
- Only intervene to keep the group focused, not to show how clever you are.
- Use questions and suggestions rather than give advice or provide answers (even where you have the answer).
- Negotiate within the group the structure and framework of processes and meetings. Most group decisions about time limits, roles, values, aims, objectives are negotiated.
- Be sensitive to the culture, beliefs and sensitivities of all in the group. This is particularly important where members belong to different ethnic groups to your own. It can also be an issue where some staff groups have different employers.
- Be flexible in the way you operate.
- Give regular encouragement by stating progress made and acknowledging achievements.
- Use humour, especially to defuse tension.
- Only intervene in group discussions when it is necessary to interrupt unhelpful behaviour.
- Monitor the energy of the group. You can expect it to dip after lunch or after a period of intense concentration. Short breaks or active exercises can help to sustain energy.

Cont

- Seek agreement from the whole group rather than using voting to reach decisions.
- If you are in doubt about whether all in the group agree – ask.
- If you don't know what to do when an intervention seems to be needed, ask the group for suggestions. Do not pretend you know everything.
- Invite feedback from the group on how the process is working.
- Encourage group skills in others – these increase the level of co-operation in a group and lead to individuals 'letting go' of their 'baggage' and identifying more with each other. People crave unity, acceptance and trust when in groups.

Hunter *et al.* (1996) also suggest various types of interventions you might use in a range of different situations when facilitating a group and a few are given in the following boxes to give you a flavour. **Note that they usually take the form of questions or suggestions to the group.**

Situations and interventions

To set the climate or the culture of the group

- How do we want to work in this group?
- What do you not want to see happening in this group?
- Which values are important?

To manage time

- How long will we spend on this issue?
- Does everyone agree?
- Let's put times beside these agenda items.

To get participation

- Let's have a round and see what everyone is thinking.
- Who would like to speak first?
- Share with the person next to you.

To maintain energy and alertness

- Energy seems to be low. There may be things holding people back. Does anyone have anything they want to say?

Cont

- Let's stand up and stretch to get the energy moving.
- Share with your partner any concerns you have on this issue.

To create the future

- What is the best way this can turn out?
- What will this lead to in three years' time?
- What do you want to end up with?

To draw out issues

- There seem to be several issues within this discussion. Let's tease them out and discuss them one at a time.
- What is the key issue here?
- Would someone like to play the role of devil's advocate here?

To keep to the task

- We are getting distracted. Let's get back on task.
- How can we move this forward?
- Who will take responsibility for carrying out this task?

To shift the level of the group

- This sounds very rational. What do people **feel** about it? (shifting from a thinking to a feeling level)
- Is everyone comfortable or do we need a break? (shifting to the physical level)

To deal with unhelpful behaviour

- Can you propose an alternative, Bob? (where Bob is blocking any new suggestions)
- Can we have one conversation at a time? (where people are whispering on the side)
- Let's separate the person from the issue here (where a personal attack is taking place).

To articulate what is not being said

- How do you account for the lack of participation in this group?
- There is something going on under the surface here. Can anyone say what it is?

Cont

To identify agreement and disagreement

- Can someone sum up what we have agreed so far?
- We do not have agreement. Let's list the different options on the flip chart.
- Who is not happy with this solution?

To encourage learning in the group

- How will you use these ideas?
- If you did this again, what would you like to be different?

Feedback

- Let's have a round of constructive criticism.
- Let's have some feedback on that idea.

Completion

- What do you need to say so that we can move on?
- What is stopping you being satisfied with the outcome?

(Hunter *et al.*, 1996)

The Practice Audit Co-ordinators were also given some tips in their training course on *how to deal with familiar 'problem' people* you may have encountered in your practice meetings.

How to deal with 'problem' people in groups

For the dominant or excessive talker

- You can establish that each member of the group contributes one idea to the discussion and must then wait until everyone else has spoken before having his or her turn again.
- When a rambling talker stops for breath, you can ask them to summarise their points so that others can comment.
- You can thank an excessive talker for their ideas and ask for the views of the rest of the group.

Cont

For the shy, withdrawn person

- Do some warm-up exercises when the group gets together.
- Talk to the person privately to find out what they are thinking.
- Direct questions to this person when you know they have particular experience or expertise on the subject being discussed.
- Do not threaten or embarrass the individual in any way.

The avoider

- Do not let conflicts remain unresolved. Keep the group working on problems until they are resolved.
- Direct questions to and elicit ideas from the avoider.
- Talk to the avoider privately to find out what is happening.

The degrader

- Set ground rules with the group at the beginning to include the rule that all ideas should be accepted without criticism. The first time someone criticises another person you must refer to this rule.
- To maintain the self-esteem of the person who is criticising, you may need to talk to him or her in private.
- Confront the persistent degrader by saying, 'you may have a point but we need to solve this problem and this isn't useful'.

The unco-operative person

- Encourage this person to explain the reasons behind his/her objection.
- Look for any aspect of their argument which supports the group's ideas to help the person move towards the majority view.
- Ask the group to deal with the individual's behaviour.

The whisperer or side conversationalist

- Stop the meeting and ask those involved to share their discussion with the group.
- Stop the meeting and comment that it is difficult to hear the discussion and concentrate with this talking going on.
- Talk to those involved in private and discuss their expectations of the meeting. If these are different from what is being covered you could suggest they leave and return at another time.
- Ask the group to deal with the behaviour.

Note: Depending on the nature of any ground rules which might have been agreed, you might be able to deal with the unhelpful behaviour by referring to them.

We have described some interventions or types of behaviour which can help your group function more effectively, whether you are an ordinary member of the group, or are working with your group to actively improve its functioning, or taking on the formal Facilitator role. There are also some specific *tools* which can help a group make progress on the road to synergy. An indication of when to use which specific tool is given on p. 40. The tools themselves are described in the following pages – however, before using a tool, bear in mind the following advice.

Planning to use tools in a group setting

When planning to use tools in a group setting it is important that:

- you understand how to use the tool
- you feel comfortable with the tool yourself
- you can explain to others the benefits of using a specific tool
- you can allay any fears about participating
- you can give explicit instructions to others
- they know what the outcome is likely to be.

Some questions to ask yourself before using tools:

- what is the purpose of using this tool?
- what will be the potential cost in terms of time, effort and resources?
- will this activity make good use of the group's time, effort and resources?
- can every person in the group see its relevance and thus be committed to it?
- what are people's concern about this activity? (It may be better to get these out into the open and address them)
- what procedures will have to be in place in order to carry out this activity?
- what will we do with the results or the outcome?

Purpose	Suggested tools
To warm up a group	*Ice breakers*
To focus on internal and external factors which will affect your new group	*Inlaws and outlaws*
To establish how a new group will operate	*Group planning template*
To review the operation of an existing group	*Clarifying the task and process of an existing group*

When groups or teams are unused to paying attention to the processes as well as the task, it will be important for you in your facilitative role to find out how they react to a different way of operating. It is useful to build in some time for *reflection* and for that reason we have enclosed the format for a simple card game that encourages participants who have been working together to reflect on how the session went.

Technique:	**Ice breakers**
Purpose:	To help create a suitable environment to achieve the goals of the meeting. Depending on the group, the purpose of the meeting, how well group members know each other already and your familiarity with the group, the prime need might be:

- to find out each other's names
- to get to know one another better
- to focus minds on the business of the day
- to express any hopes and fears about what might happen that day
- to become mentally alert.

Tips for use:

- Be clear about what is the primary need of the group at the start of the meeting or activity.
- Select an ice breaker which best meets the needs of the group.
- Keep it simple and short, particularly if the group is large.
- Be sensitive to how the ice breaker might affect participants.

Materials required: Simple instructions given verbally or written on a flip chart or overhead.
Alternative: a set of cards for ice breakers where the activity involves participants answering a question.

There are many examples of ice breakers in training manuals. The following are a selection which have proved acceptable in primary care settings locally.

Adjectival Annie

A light-hearted ice breaker which allows participants to learn each other's names. Each member of the group in turn states their Christian name, prefixed by an adjective beginning with the same letter as their name, and which best describes them. For example, 'Hi, I am zany Zelda'. A useful variation when you are working with an established group as an outsider, is to ask each member to describe the person on their right using one word only. This usually generates some hilarity in the group.

What have you left behind?

Suggest to the group that they each think of a mental obstacle linked to home or work which might interfere with their full participation in the group – is the ironing left undone, does the grass need cutting, do those patient notes need to be updated? Whatever it might be, suggest that they give themselves permission to set it aside for today. Share your own thoughts with the group, and ask if anyone else would like to do the same.

Get up and move around

Physical activity centred round a requirement to mingle with others can help overcome initial reticence to participate in the group, a feeling of sluggishness at the start of the day or after a heavy meal. You can suggest that the group forms a line in order of height, shoe size or birthday. To make it harder you can outlaw speaking.

Express hopes, wishes and concerns

It may aid participation if all members are given an opportunity to express their feelings about taking part. You can prepare in advance a number of cards, each with one question on it, and ask each member to select one from the pack. Questions might include:

- What do I most dread about today?
- What do I hope we will achieve today?
- What will help us get the job done today?

The members of the group, in turn, read out their question and give their answer.

Technique:	**Inlaws and outlaws**

Purpose:
- Useful for a new group.
- To focus on internal and external influences on the group.
- To separate these categories in order to develop workable relationships with them.

Tips for use:
- Start the discussion by posing the general question, 'How do others affect our success as a group?'
- Follow up by asking specifically, 'What *insider* influences are there on our group, e.g. systems, resources, patients/clients, colleagues in other teams within our organisation?' These are noted as being 'Inlaws'.
- And then, 'What *outsider* influences are there, e.g. laws, obligations, other organisations, external resources, society?' These are 'Outlaws'.
- Use a round or brainstorming to generate as many ideas as possible (*see* Chapter 5).
- Volunteers note on the flip charts all ideas as 'Inlaws' or 'Outlaws'.
- After the supply of ideas has been exhausted ask, 'What can we live with?' and 'What can we change?'
- Complete the following matrix on your chart.

Suggest that seeing factors which influence them in this way is the beginning of developing a plan for dealing with them.

Materials required:
Three flip charts: one each for the volunteers and one for the facilitator.

Adapted from Nilson, 1993.

Inlaws and outlaws

INLAWS (live with)	INLAWS (change)
OUTLAWS (live with)	**OUTLAWS** (change)

Technique:	**Planning for a small group**
Purpose:	To provide a focus and some guidelines for a new group when planning how it will operate, before it launches into its task.
Tips for use:	• You may need to sell the idea of using this tool to the group in question as it will take perhaps half an hour out of the first meeting. You can facilitate this discussion as a member of the group or as an external Facilitator.
	• You can use a number of facilitative techniques alongside the tool, e.g. an ice breaker, brainstorming, a round (*see* Chapter 5).
	• It may also help the group if you employ some interventions such as drawing out quiet members, seeking agreement after discussion, airing worries or concerns.
	• The group may not be able to answer all the questions without consulting some other person or authority. This may be a good thing as lack of clarity often hinders the work of sub-groups which have been appointed by the main group to work on a specific task.
	• You may want to revisit these questions after a period of time or use *Clarifying the task and process of an existing group* tool.
Materials required:	• A copy of the questions shown on p. 46, for each member of the group.
	• A flip chart to note content of discussion.
	• A résumé of the discussion and a record of decisions made which will then act as the operating framework for the group.

Planning for a small group

Some questions to guide discussion and
decision making on how a group will operate

1   What is the role of this group? (remit, authority)

2   What do we think we ought to be doing? (objectives)

3   When and where are we going to meet? (venue, timetable, suitable to
    participants, will allow us to complete the task)

4   How are we going to work together in the group? (procedures, decision-
    making techniques)

5   Do we need a group leader/co-ordinator? (alternative ways of working)

6   What do we want to avoid doing?

7   Do we want to have any ground rules for the way we operate? (attendance,
    commitment, helpful behaviour, dealing with conflicting views)

8   What are the reporting arrangements? (do we need minutes, who will do
    them, what will be in them, who gets them?)

Technique:	**Clarifying the task and process of an existing group**
Purpose:	For use in an existing group where members have acknowledged that they are not working together either productively or harmoniously. It provides the opportunity to review systematically the culture and working processes of the group and can stimulate discussion as to where changes might be made.
Tips for use:	• Define the purpose of using the tool. You might want to include some reference to the theoretical benefits of working in a group (*see* p. 18) and the elements of task and process.
	• Outline any benefits which might result from addressing the questions.
	• Describe how the tool works.
	• Obtain the agreement of the group to use it.

The questions listed in the table can be addressed in a number of ways. For example, small groups might take one section each. Alternatively, the Facilitator could pose each question to the whole group for open discussion. You might prefer to issue a questionnaire containing the questions, collate the results and structure a discussion around your findings.

As always, it is preferable to highlight, discuss and address *issues* rather than pinpoint or attack *individuals*. Any proposals for change in the group culture or working processes should be discussed fully and agreed by the group itself.

Following any changes made to existing working practices, *review* the situation after an appropriate period of time, using the same technique.

Materials required:	• Flip chart to record main discussion/decisions (optional).
	• Questionnaire based on list of questions on p. 48 (optional).
	• Documentation of any decisions made about change in ways of working.

Clarifying the task and process of an existing group

Some questions to guide discussion and decision making on how a group will operate

Goals

- Are we all here for a common purpose?
- What is our task in this group?
- Do we need to revise our goals?
- How will we know when we have completed our task?

Roles

- Is the composition of the group appropriate?
- Who does what in this group?
- Is everyone clear about their own role?
- Is everyone clear about others' roles?
- Are we each able to fulfil our role?
- Can any constraints to carrying out our roles be reduced?

Procedures

- Do we meet often enough to achieve our aims?
- Do we waste time?
- Do we make it easier for everyone to contribute their ideas and opinions or do we let one or two do all the talking?
- Does everyone feel comfortable about challenging statements made in the group?
- Do we handle conflict effectively in the group?
- Do we make sure we have all the appropriate information available before making decisions?
- Do we specify who will implement any decisions?
- Do we follow up decisions and review the outcome?

Relationships

- How is morale within the group?
- Are we sensitive to how other people are feeling?
- Can we tolerate failure and give support rather than blame?

Technique: **Reflections card game**

Purpose: When groups or teams are unused to paying attention to the *processes* of working together, it is important to find out how they react to a different way of operating. It is useful to build some time for *reflection* into an away day or other group session. This simple card game encourages participants who have been working together to think about how the session went.

Tips for use: In essence, each person takes a card from a pile in the centre of the table, thinks of a word or phrase to complete the statement, then reads the whole statement out loud to the group. A list of possible statements appears on p. 50.

You can vary the content of the statements to suit your own purposes. If you laminate the cards they will be more durable.

The answers can form part of an evaluation of the session and, as such, can give valuable information to aid the planning of any similar event. The activity also allows individuals to express any feelings they have within the group rather than leaving the setting and talking about them somewhere less appropriate.

Reflections card game

- The thing that surprised me most about today was . . .

- Something I'm glad we talked about today was . . .

- Something I wish we could have talked about today was . . .

- The most important thing I learned about today was . . .

- The most interesting thing I learned about today was . . .

- The thing I enjoyed least about today was . . .

- The person I learned something new about today was . . .

- The thing I was least surprised about today was . . .

- The thing I wish we had spent more time on today was . . .

- The thing that frustrated me most today was . . .

- The person I would have liked to have heard more from today was . . .

- The best moment for me today was . . .

- The thing that made me most anxious today was . . .

- The first thing I will do as a result of today is . . .

- The funniest thing for me today was . . .

- The thing that pleased me most about today was . . .

- The thing I was dreading most about today was . . .

We move on now to discuss a particular facet of working with others in a group – **Meetings** – and how to make them more effective. Before we do that, read and reflect now on what facilitation was able to achieve in 15 practices, scattered throughout a whole Scottish Health Board region.

Case Study 5
Facilitation skills, qualities and effects
The FED Project

An external educational facilitator worked with 15 practices on an educational project over a two-year period, helping them identify areas for development within the practice and providing resources and support to begin the development process (Duffy, Griffin and Bain, 1998). The project was driven by the practices which made use of training, advice, help and group facilitation as and when it suited them.

At the end of two years, representatives from the practices were asked what qualities they had felt were vital in the Facilitator. The following paragraph from the project report summarises their replies:

'The background of the Facilitator should be relevant to the context of primary care, and be evident in an understanding of the pressures of work and the dynamics of primary healthcare teams. The Facilitator is of benefit to a practice in his/her neutrality, objectivity, honesty, empathy, sensitivity, contextual knowledge, reliability, openness, and positive approach . . .'

This type of approach had allowed the project to provide the practices with:

- a **catalyst** for change
- **insight** to the organisation on its strengths and weaknesses and unique identity
- **increased awareness** of the value of teamwork, good communication and effective management of information in providing patient care
- **help** in assessing its needs and establishing its priorities for development
- **facilitation** of the production of the practice development plan by giving guidance on its structure and content

- a **kick-start** to the development process where practices did not know where and how to begin
- **encouragement** toward wider and more equal participation amongst the practice team in developing the practice
- presentation of a **positive, constructive approach** to practice development planning
- provision of **objective and impartial evidence** which could justify some major change
- the **nurturing** of skills and confidence.

Chapter 5

Making meetings more effective

Summary

In the theory section of this chapter we discuss:

- *meetings as an effective means of communication*
- *formal and informal meetings*
- *the purpose of meetings*
- *the terms of reference of a meeting*
- *characteristics of an effective meeting*
- *convening and chairing a successful meeting*
- *reasons for disillusionment with meetings*
- *decision making in meetings*
- *problem solving in meetings.*

We then look at meetings in general practice and describe:

- *the variety of meetings commonly held*
- *particular problems associated with practice meetings.*

We suggest that you can help your practice meetings become more effective by:

- *setting up any new meetings in a more efficient way*
- *reviewing existing meetings to see how effective they are*
- *encouraging the chairperson to look at guidelines for convening and chairing meetings.*

We describe some techniques for:

- *identifying problems*
- *thinking creatively*
- *reaching consensus.*

Theory

Meetings can be an effective means of communication in a number of circumstances:

- to meet an individual's need to receive and contribute information
- to obtain a range of views
- to create a broader base for implementing decisions
- to reach better quality decisions
- to encourage unity of thought and action
- to serve the process of democratic management
- to build morale.

It is usual to distinguish between formal and informal meetings, although in real life these tend to be the two ends of a scale.

Formal meetings

These are highly structured and usually have the following characteristics:

- notice is given of the date of the meeting
- a pre-arranged agenda is followed
- standard meeting procedures are adhered to
- items are discussed in the form of motions and amendments
- discussion is controlled by a chairperson and all contributions are addressed to him/her
- proceedings are recorded in the form of minutes.

Informal meetings

These, on the other hand, are less governed by procedure and may have the following characteristics:

- they may be arranged at short notice
- there may be only one topic for discussion and there may be no formal agenda
- theoretically there are no restrictions on what is said or done
- discussion is controlled by the dynamics of the group
- there are no formal roles, procedures or documentation involved.

Most meetings in the workplace fall somewhere between the two extremes.

The purpose of meetings

A more useful distinction to be made relates to the purpose or function of meetings. Some meetings take place in order to *share information*, while others are designed for *problem solving* and *decision making*. In the interests of efficiency it is often preferable to keep these two types of meeting separate. It has been suggested that, if an issue arises at an information meeting that requires problem solving it is advisable to postpone it until the next decision-making meeting (Porritt, 1990). Likewise, too much time spent in briefing members at a problem-solving meeting may mean that no decisions are reached. If meetings are designed to fulfil both functions, then it may be useful when compiling the agenda to keep information items separate from problem-solving items.

Any type of meeting benefits from a systematic approach to its organisation; a positive attitude on the part of the participants; and some time and effort spent on getting the procedures right, particularly the procedures for making decisions, and ensuring that these are implemented.

Terms of reference for a meeting

These determine what a group (or committee) can and cannot do. Awareness of the specific terms of reference can prevent some of the frustrations and dissatisfaction caused by the feeling that a meeting is not achieving very much or that the group is powerless. Even if the terms of reference are not formally written down, everyone in the group should be aware of the following points:

- the role of the group
- its precise function
- its limitations
- to whom it is responsible
- who is responsible to it.

Since all organisations are dynamic and the terms of reference will evolve or be altered over time, it is important to make sure that everyone involved is aware of any changes. For a single meeting, its objectives (or goals) are its terms of reference. For any meeting a clear statement of its objectives will encourage all discussion and energy to be directed towards achieving these. It helps if objectives are SMART:

Specific   The wording should leave no doubt about what is required.

Measurable   The goal or objective should be readily measurable, and the results should be available quickly and regularly.

Attainable   If the goal offers poor chances of success then it becomes a demotivating force.

Relevant   Goals must be seen to be relevant to the goals of both the organisation and the individual.

Timebound   How much and how soon must be spelt out – otherwise the goal is little more than a 'wish'.

An **effective meeting** might be characterised by the following:

Characteristics of an effective meeting

- An informal comfortable atmosphere.
- Clearly understood and accepted objectives.
- All discussion and energy directed towards achieving those objectives.
- Members who treat each other as people and don't show indifference to each other.
- Communication patterns marked by openness, allowing full discussion and participation by all.
- A strong, but not autocratic leadership.
- A shared understanding of appropriate and helpful behaviour.
- Effective decision making and problem solving.

A **Chairperson** and **Secretary** are usually appointed where a group meets on a regular basis. While all in attendance can contribute to the success of a meeting, the role of the Chairperson or meeting leader is crucial, with the Secretary often sharing some of the important preparation and follow-up duties.

Convening and chairing a successful meeting

Five specific stages are typically described for convening and chairing a successful meeting:

1 planning
2 opening the meeting
3 managing the business
4 closing the meeting
5 following-up the meeting.

Convening and chairing a successful meeting

1 Planning

- Deciding if a meeting is really required or if there is some other mechanism for seeking ideas or achieving agreement.
- Identifying the purpose and agreeing realistic objectives.
- Formulating an effective agenda which should lead to achieving objectives.
- Ensuring that the right people with knowledge, expertise, interest and power are invited to attend.
- Ensuring that all necessary documents are produced and distributed where required, in advance.
- Checking that the venue is suitably equipped in every way and will encourage full participation.
- Preparing oneself mentally and physically to lead the meeting to a successful outcome.
- Developing some contingency plans if things go wrong.

2 Opening the meeting

- Creating a positive first impression.
- Starting the meeting on time.
- Welcoming people, clarifying roles and responsibilities if necessary.
- Focusing on what the meeting must achieve.
- Establishing ground rules and enforcing them.
- Gaining commitment to the agenda.
- Agreeing use of time and when the meeting will end.
- Dealing with any 'housekeeping' issues.

3 Managing the business

- Steering discussion in a logical, structured way.
- Concentrating on managing the process.
- Using problem-solving techniques to work through complex issues.
- Managing time so that agenda items receive the appropriate level of discussion.
- Ensuring the meeting ends on time.
- Encouraging full and active participation by all.
- Handling conflict.
- Summarising to confirm agreement and ownership of action points.
- Ensuring that notes record key agreements, facts or opinions or verbatim quotes.

Cont

4 Closing the meeting

- Summarising the key points – who will do what and by when?
- Clarifying how outstanding issues will be resolved.
- Confirming arrangements for follow-up documentation.
- Agreeing details for the next meeting, if any.
- Thanking everyone for their contribution.
- Leaving the place tidy.

5 Following-up the meeting

- Reviewing the effectiveness of the meeting and identifying opportunities for improvement.
- Reviewing the action points and developing implementation plans.
- Actively following-up progress on action points.
- Ensuring timely distribution of minutes or other papers.
- Maintaining support of key participants by keeping them informed of progress.
- Preparing for the next meeting.

(Bray, 1995)

Disillusionment with meetings

Unfortunately many people express disillusionment about the usefulness of meetings. Here are two typical quotes about meetings:

'A meeting is a group of people who keep minutes and waste hours.'

'A meeting brings together a group of the unfit, appointed by the unwilling, to do the unnecessary, for the ungrateful.'

The reasons for this cynicism can usually be related to one or more of the Four Ps – **P**reparation, **P**urpose, **P**eople and **P**lace. Examples of frustrations might include:

Preparation
- The agenda arrived late or not at all.
- The chairperson was poorly prepared.
- The meeting was arranged for an inconvenient time.

Purpose
- The purpose of the meeting was unclear.
- The meeting was unnecessary.
- No clear objectives were agreed.

People
- The wrong people were present, or the right people absent.
- Those present were not committed to the group and its objectives.
- Nothing was decided.

Place
- The venue was too small.
- The seating made discussion difficult.
- There were frequent interruptions from phone calls.

Some of these frustrations are illustrated in this next case study of a practice meeting in another city centre practice whose patients were drawn mainly from deprived areas. Note how individual needs tend to overshadow group needs.

Case Study 6
The Pink Practice Meeting

Dr Black (Female) Senior partner in 50s, forceful and autocratic. Very interested in practice profit, but making no input on falling list size and increasing costs. Chairs the meeting.

Dr White (Female) Mid 40s. Three-quarter time, interested in patient care but slow to embrace change. Talkative and wanders off the subject often. Trainer for GP Registrar.

Dr Brown (Male) 40s. Very hard working but not interested in administration unless it has a direct impact on what he does. Dour and irritable, heading for burnout, but cannot see it coming. May be late for the meeting – out on house calls.

Dr Orange (Female) Late 40s. Aware of major problems in practice management, but cannot manage to get anything to change. Very popular with patients, and staff find her approachable but she is a little shy.

Dr Green (Male) Early 30s. Joined the practice three years ago as it was the only job going. Not impressed with older partners' clinical skills. Feels there is a lack of teamwork and efficiency.

Mrs Grey   Practice Manager, 40 years old. Frustrated and irritable – feels she hasn't been given the freedom to introduce change.

Miss Blues   Senior Receptionist, 30 years old. Obstructive – feels that change will involve more work for her and staff. Puts her own slant on minutes.

An observer at the practice meeting noted the following:

- Dr Green appeared five minutes late, and proceeded to finish off some patient notes.
- Dr Orange arrived 10 minutes later.
- Dr Brown turned up after the meeting had finished.
- The minutes were not ready in time for the meeting.
- The table was littered with journals.
- The first item on the agenda was the brand of coffee the practice ought to buy. There was considerable heated discussion on this point. A decision was deferred.
- Dr Black wanted an instant decision on how to pay the tax shortfall – no-one had seen the up-to-date figures until that moment and no decision was taken. Mrs Grey to 'look into it'.
- Dr White indulged in a nostalgic 'ramble' about the good old days.
- Dr Green made a unilateral decision about a new prescribing policy, ignoring mutterings of disagreement from colleagues.
- Dr Black presented an item on partner workload, proposed by Dr Brown who was still out on house calls, but as he did not have all the information there was much speculative discussion but no decision made about what to do next.
- Miss Blues made coffee and answered a phone call, thus missing out on several points for the minutes. She clattered the cups and saucers, disturbing the meeting.
- Mrs Grey and Miss Blues began a side conversation on possible changes to appointment times. Throughout the meeting Mrs Grey showed her frustration with the partners.
- Dr White tried in vain to press the point that the practice might lose their training status but the Chairman dismissed her concerns and suggested she do a patch up job as she did two years ago for the reapproval visit.
- Dr Orange left early before the close of business – quickly followed by Dr Green.
- No date was set for the next meeting.

Decision making in meetings

In decision-making meetings, the purpose of group decision making is to decide upon well-considered, well-understood realistic action towards goals every member wants to achieve. A group decision implies that some agreement prevails among group members as to which course of action, among the many possible, is most suitable and desirable for achieving the group's goals.

There are five major characteristics of an effective decision:

1 the resources of the group are fully realised
2 time is well used
3 the decision is correct or of high quality
4 the decision is implemented fully by all the group members
5 the problem-solving ability of the group is enhanced or at least not lessened.
(Johnson and Johnson, 1991)

Some groups have difficulty making decisions where members do not agree on what the decision should be.

There are many ways a group can make a decision and each method has its uses and is appropriate under certain circumstances. Each also has particular consequences for the group.

Methods of decision making

According to Johnson and Johnson (1991) there are seven major methods of decision making, each with its own inherent advantages and disadvantages.

Methods of making a decision in a group		
Technique	**Advantage**	**Disadvantage**
1 Decision by authority without discussion – e.g. leader makes decision without consulting the group members)	Quick; useful for simple, routine decisions	Not all the group may understand, agree and/or want to implement the decisions; quality of decision dependent on expertise of only one person

Cont

Technique	Advantage	Disadvantage
2 Decision by expert – group allows the most expert member decide what the group will do	Quick; useful when implementation does not involve all the group members	How to tell which group member has the most expertise may be affected by popularity or personal power; group may not be committed to implementing the decision
3 Decision by averaging individuals' opinions – chairperson asks for each individual's opinion, no discussion takes place	Members are consulted; can be time saving; better than **1** but usually less effective than **2**	Commitment to decision may not be strong; some expert opinion may be annulled by least knowledgeable opinion
4 Decision by authority after group discussion – leader makes decision after full discussion with group	The benefits of group discussion improve accuracy of leader's decision	Members may try to impress leader or tell him/her what they think he/she wants to hear
5 Decision by minority – executive group or working party appointed with decision-making powers	Can be an efficient use of time; useful where member involvement in implementation not required	Majority may not be committed to the decision; some may be reticent about expressing their disagreement

Cont

Technique	Advantage	Disadvantage
6 **Decision by majority vote** – almost taken for granted as the natural way to make decisions	Useful where commitment by all is not essential	Encourages 'winners' and 'losers'; may create sabotage sub-groups
7 **Decision by consensus** – collective opinion arrived at in a climate which allows full participation and influence by all members	All members understand decision and support decision; can produce innovative creative and high-quality decisions	Takes time, energy and individual skill; not suitable where emergency exists

Which decision-making method to choose?

An effective group understands each method of decision making well enough to choose the method which is best for:

- the type of decision to be made
- the amount of time and resources available
- the history of the group
- the type of task being worked on
- the kind of climate the group wishes to establish
- the type of environment in which the group is working.

Where a group is engaged in collective decision making there is a recognisable procedure, known as the **'rational decision process'** involving the following stages:

- analysing the situation
- defining the problem

- identifying the goals
- establishing the priorities
- generating alternative solutions
- identifying criteria for evaluating those alternative solutions
- evaluating alternative solutions
- selecting the 'best' solution.

As we have already suggested, decision making occurs within the context of problem solving. Some factors that help and hinder effective problem solving are provided in the following boxes.

Factors which aid effective problem solving

- A well-structured group.
- Time to exchange views and debate ideas.
- Individual accountability by members for doing their share of the work.
- Individual members with developed group skills.
- Opportunity to review how well the group is functioning.
- Agreement on where group should be.
- Creative and divergent reasoning to come up with alternative solutions.

Factors which hinder effective problem solving

- Inadequate definition of the problem.
- A critical, competitive or evaluative climate.
- Inadequate motivation to solve the problem.
- Poor communication within the group.
- Failure to identify proper alternative courses of action.
- Poor evaluation of alternative solutions.

(Johnson and Johnson, 1991)

> ## General Practice

The need for meetings

At the GP 97 Conference, Lyn Longridge, a practice management consultant, said:

> *'One thing of which you can be sure is that the need for meetings in general practice will not diminish. The only way to avoid the worst effects of having change imposed on you, is to be prepared for it. Forward planning is essential and the way to achieve this is to brainstorm, consult, discuss and make decisions. It is particularly important that you [as Practice Manager] are able to run effective meetings within your practice where all these activities can take place within a structured framework.'*

The variety of practice meetings

In general practice, a variety of meetings involving participation by many different combinations of people such as GPs, Practice Nurses, Community Nursing staff and Administrative staff need to take place at different intervals. The practice, as a 'business', needs to be managed. The partners need to meet regularly with the practice management staff to ensure that the practice runs smoothly and efficiently. It is considered good practice to hold meetings with all staff present and to involve them in the decisions which directly affect them. At clinical meetings doctors and nursing staff will discuss disease management, protocols for care and any changes in established procedures. Informal meetings may take place daily between nursing staff and doctors on individual patient care. An Audit Co-ordinator may run audit meetings from time to time to encourage involvement in the process and feedback results. Meetings of the whole primary healthcare team, or representatives of it, involving attached and visiting members as well as employed staff, may take place to decide the shape of the Practice Development Plan or similar long-range strategy document.

Features of meetings in general practice

Time is in short supply for all those working in general practice. It is vital that meetings are productive and that decisions are both made *and* implemented. The common complaints about meetings (*see* p. 55) all apply. Importantly, in general practice, there are some particular factors to deal with:

- doctors and management staff may lack the skills to manage meetings, yet they are normally required to take on that role

- the chairperson may be appointed based on status rather than skill
- the nature of the daily work means that it is difficult for all the relevant people to attend all the relevant meetings
- some more junior staff may be inhibited because of the hierarchy within the practice
- change happens so fast that decisions may have to be made sometimes without adequate consultation and discussion
- it can be difficult to find a suitable meeting place within a practice.

You might also, at this stage, want to review what was said about working in groups in general practice (*see* Chapter 4).

So how can you help to make meetings run more smoothly?

In the following sections, we look at how to improve practice meetings through effective planning and chairing, how to diagnose what is going wrong with your practice meetings, and how to improve problem solving and decision making.

Facilitate Your Own Practice

Facilitating the planning and review of practice meetings

As described in previous sections, you can behave in practice meetings in a generally more facilitative way while still in your normal role – using techniques like offering information, seeking ideas, supporting others in their views, monitoring standards.

When a **new group** begins to meet you can suggest that they follow the guidelines for small groups – establishing the role of the group; its objectives; the practical details of venue/membership/timetable; agree procedures, ground rules for behaviour and participation; reporting arrangements.

It might also help your practice meeting if you can interest your colleagues in **reviewing** how effective your meetings are. For this purpose we have included a **Meetings Checklist** that all those commonly attending the meetings complete, and which forms the basis of some discussion of how the situation can be improved.

If there is a regular chairperson you might suggest to him/her that you look together at the **Five Stages of Convening and Chairing Meetings** shown on p. 57.

Problems sometimes occur in practices where a key role is not filled by the mix of skills and personalities attending meetings. Here is how the Brown Practice, a four partner seaside practice, identified the cause of most of their bright ideas for development failing to come to fruition.

Case Study 7
The Brown Practice Meetings

The Brown Practice had a regular calendar of practice meetings. The whole practice met every quarter; the individual staff groups met formally once a month and liaised informally on a daily basis; the practice management group convened fortnightly; and the clinical staff met formally on a weekly basis.

There seemed to be a perennial problem in all the groups – the members generated lots of ideas but few of them came to fruition. In addition, the practice was enthusiastic about taking part in almost every new initiative which came along. When they did take stock at an away day many people commented that they felt the practice 'took on too much' and that in spite of all these meetings some situations never seemed to change.

Two of the practice team attended a local workshop on meetings skills and were introduced to the Belbin Self-Perception Inventory which identified roles that individuals tend to adopt in meetings.* Belbin's observations include: a mix of types is preferable and where some key roles are absent in a group, the members have to try actively to fill that gap by modifying their behaviour to some extent. The two Brown Practice representatives took copies of the Inventory back to the practice and all the team filled them in. They were intrigued to find that their practice team lacked both a *completer/finisher* and a *monitor/evaluator* but abounded in *plants, team workers* and *resource investigators*. Having identified the gaps, the team could understand better why plans failed to materialise and could also resolve to pay more attention to those aspects of groupworking.

(Your local Department of General Practice may hold a licence for the use of *Interplace*. Alternatively, you can contact Belbin Associates direct for more details.)

---

* Belbin Associates' *Interplace*, 3–4 Bennel Court, West Street, Comberton, Cambridge, CB3 7DS

Using Belbin to explain problems in your practice

It may be that you recognise *your* practice in one of the following examples. Belbin might have an explanation for your problem.

Typical problem	Possible reason
Underachieving	Needs *co-ordinator* or *completer/finisher* to ensure task is completed
Team with conflict	Needs *team worker* to resolve difficulties
Mediocre performance	Needs *shaper* to generate innovative ideas and/or *resource investigator* to identify skills and resources within and outwith the team
Makes mistakes	Needs *monitor/evaluator* to encourage the team to think things through and check the quality of their decisions

With problem solving and decision making being central to the purpose of most meetings, the next section suggests some tools to aid these processes.

Tips and Tools

We have already described some useful tools.

Purpose	Suggested tool
To establish how a new group will run its meetings	*Planning for a small group*
To improve the planning for and chairing of practice meetings	*Convening a successful meeting*

In the following pages we introduce you to some more tools and techniques:

Purpose	Suggested tool
To diagnose problems in the functioning of your practice meetings	*The Meetings Checklist*
To solve problems by identifying their roots	*Root Cause Analysis* *The Five Whys*
To stimulate creative thinking	*Brainstorming*
To encourage wider participation	*A round*
To make decisions by consensus	*Guidelines for reaching consensus*

To diagnose problems in your practice meetings you might suggest that your group use *The Meetings Checklist* (*see* p. 74). This checklist asks group members to rate the extent to which common meetings problems occur in their own group and compare that to other groups of which they have experience.

Identifying the roots of a problem

In order to solve a problem it is obviously necessary to establish the factors which are creating the problem or are part of it. Here are two useful tools and real life examples of their use.

Root Cause Analysis

Root Cause Analysis is a way of tracing a problem situation back to its real roots and identifying what needs to be addressed in order to alleviate the problem.

The problem situation is displayed in a shaded oval, e.g. (**Low morale**), and the contributory factors appear as side shoots of the root system or as a sequence from problem-to-root cause. The Grey Practice was experiencing pervasive low morale and Root Cause Analysis suggested a possible reason for it.

Root cause analysis of low morale in The Grey Practice

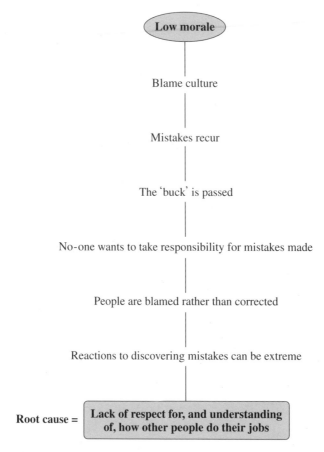

Low morale

Blame culture

Mistakes recur

The 'buck' is passed

No-one wants to take responsibility for mistakes made

People are blamed rather than corrected

Reactions to discovering mistakes can be extreme

Root cause = **Lack of respect for, and understanding of, how other people do their jobs**

Case Study 8 describes the process by which the root cause was identified and communicated back to the practice by an external Facilitator.

Case Study 8
Analysis of low morale in The Grey Practice

The Grey Practice was experiencing widespread low morale, particularly amongst the administrative staff. Attempts had been made to establish the exact cause of this general feeling but some staff had felt unwilling to express their views in a whole-practice away day held some months previously. No-one knew what to do to try to remedy the situation.

An external Facilitator was invited in to speak with all staff on a range of issues relevant to the organisation and management of the practice. In one-to-one interviews she encouraged all staff to feel relaxed and comfortable about discussing some difficult areas, in the knowledge that their views would be kept confidential and the feedback report would not identify individuals within the practice, but would rather concentrate on common themes and suggestions for improvement.

The Facilitator did indeed find that there were problems of low morale. She heard of factions within the practice, loss of confidence among some staff, an unwillingness to work for each other and a general feeling that this was causing upset and even ill health for many people within the practice. A culture of blame was also observed. It was a difficult scenario to feed back, requiring sensitivity and respect from the Facilitator in her report, without skirting around the key issues that would have to be addressed if the situation were to improve.

The Facilitator used Root Cause Analysis to try to get to the real cause of low morale. She presented her ideas in diagrammatic form (*see* p. 70) which allowed the concepts to be seen at a glance and also removed the need to express challenging ideas in paragraphs of text that might make rather depressing reading. The whole practice attended a feedback meeting where the concepts were again presented. The Facilitator was relieved to learn that those attending did indeed accept her findings and could cope with them being aired in public in this way.

The Five Whys

'The Five Whys' is another technique for tracing a problem back to its roots through asking the question 'why?' as often as it takes to get to a point where the real root has been identified and the question will no longer provide an answer.

In The Silver Practice, the Practice Manager helped her administrative staff identify the real cause for the delay in entering test results on to the new medical records computer programme.

Case Study 9
Use of 'The Five Whys' in The Silver Practice

Q 'Why are the test results piling up in the tray towards the end of the week?'
A 'Because there is no-one here to put them on the computer on a Thursday.'

Q 'But why is that – only Mary is off that day.'
A 'Nobody else has the time.'

Q 'But why is that?'
A 'Because that leaves only Linda and Margaret, and Linda needs to help Margaret with the claims forms on a Thursday.'

Q 'Why can't Margaret do them all herself – there is plenty of time.'
A 'She needs Linda to check them first before she sends them out.'

Q 'Why is that necessary?'
A 'Actually, she got a few wrong last month and is not confident about doing them herself.'

Q 'Why did she get them wrong?'
A 'She was only shown a couple of times and didn't quite grasp it all.'

The real cause for the delay in entering test results on to the new medical records computer programme is Margaret's loss of confidence in successfully completing the claims form. The answer is to give her some extra training in that task.

To stimulate creative thinking

We said earlier that *creative thinking* helps a group reach a good decision. *Brainstorming* is a useful technique and can help to generate a variety of ideas in a short time, and produce new and creative ideas. Specific instructions for three types of brainstorming are included at the end of this chapter.

To encourage wider participation in discussion

Participation in group discussion can be unequal or variable, as highlighted earlier when we discussed the effects of status. It may be helpful if the Facilitator states the issue or the problem and invites everyone in a group to say something one by one in a systematic way – in 'a round'. See the end of this chapter for more details.

To make decisions by consensus

Decision making in general practice takes many forms – the seven main techniques were described on pp. 61–3. Increasingly, practices are trying to reach *consensus* decisions on issues where the impact of the decision will be felt by many in the practice, and where the successful implementation is dependent on the commitment of the majority of the practice team members. True consensus means that everyone agrees what the decision should be. Achieving consensus can be time consuming as an ideal but it is useful if participants understand the factors that can help a group reach consensus and so display helpful behaviour. In that way a decision can be agreed on by the whole group so that each individual feels s/he has had a real opportunity to influence that decision.

In facilitating your practice, you can begin the process by discussing what consensus means and referring your group to the following guidelines for reaching consensus.

Guidelines for reaching consensus

- Take time to learn what each member knows that could help solve the problem.
- Present your own opinions logically and clearly.
- Avoid arguing blindly for your opinions.
- Listen to others' reactions and consider them carefully.
- Avoid changing your mind just for the sake of reaching agreement or to avoid conflict. Support only solutions with which you at least partly agree.
- Avoid conflict-reducing procedures such as tossing a coin or voting – these do not lead to consensus.
- Accept differences of opinion as natural and healthy and leading ultimately to better quality decisions.
- If stalemate is reached, do not assume that some must win and others lose. Look for the next most acceptable alternative for all concerned.
- Strive to create and maintain a climate where everyone feels comfortable and motivated to express his/her opinions.

Technique:	<div align="center">**Meetings checklist**</div>
Purpose:	To review the operation of any group meetings with particular reference to the progress of discussion and decision making. Allows some comparison between the particular meetings in question and meetings in general, relative to the experiences of those completing the checklist.
Tips for use:	<ul><li>Explain the benefits of using this tool to gain acceptance of it, e.g. it might help address the issue that time is always short and that meetings are not fully productive. If the group could identify problem areas and address them, it could perhaps become more effective in meetings.</li><li>Ensure that all those completing it realise that there are two ratings to be given – one for meetings in general and the other for their particular group meetings.</li><li>Some of the questions may appear quite threatening. People will feel more comfortable if checklists are completed on an anonymous basis and the results collated.</li><li>Explain what will happen with the results so that everyone is clear about what the next step will be.</li><li>As a general principle, it is better to concentrate on the issue rather than individuals. Having identified key problem areas with the group, concentrate then on how to improve rather than blame individuals. Ways of improving might include setting and referring to ground rules; employing facilitative interventions; appointing an observer for the next meeting whose role it is to flag up the occurrence of a particular fault so that the incident can be discussed.</li><li>There may be some faults with your particular group which do not appear on the checklist. In order that the full picture is revealed and discussed, you might want to use a *silent brainstorm* (p. 78) to seek suggestions for any additions to be made to the checklist.</li></ul>

Instructions for completion

The following weaknesses or failures frequently impede the progress of discussion and decision making in meetings. So that your group can identify and discuss its particular problem areas and generate solutions, rate each item on a scale of 0–5, where:

0 = the problem is irrelevant in this group's meetings
1 = the fault hardly occurs at all
5 = the fault is evident most of the time.

- In **column A** give your rating for your **own** particular group.
- In **column B** give your rating of how typical, in your experience, each particular fault is for **meetings generally**.

Results will be collated and overall feedback given to the group.

Problem area	A	B
1 Failure to listen to what other members have to say	☐	☐
2 Constantly re-iterating arguments	☐	☐
3 Constantly interrupting	☐	☐
4 Trying to put others down	☐	☐
5 Failure to participate	☐	☐
6 Silent members not drawn in	☐	☐
7 Dominant members allowed to dominate	☐	☐
8 Everyone putting their own views rather than clarifying and developing and encouraging others' views	☐	☐
9 Raising irrelevant or unhelpful points	☐	☐
10 Unwillingness to compromise	☐	☐
11 Dismissing others' ideas without proper discussion	☐	☐
12 Not recognising how others are feeling	☐	☐
13 Concentrating on making a good impression rather than on getting the task completed	☐	☐
14 Disturbing the process with private conversations	☐	☐
15 Not listening or paying attention	☐	☐
16 Not following agreed procedures or plans	☐	☐
17 Not completing agreed tasks	☐	☐
18 Not attending agreed meetings	☐	☐
19 Not paying attention to the time	☐	☐
20 Not being clear about what has been decided	☐	☐
21 Not being clear about who will do what has been decided	☐	☐
22 Not reviewing progress of plans made previously	☐	☐

Technique:	**Brainstorming**
Purpose:	• To generate a wide variety of ideas in a short space of time. • To produce novel or creative ideas.
Tips for use:	• Write the problem or topic where all members of the group can see it – on a flip chart for example. • Encourage expression of all ideas, however zany. • Make sure that everyone understands that no judgements should be made about the quality of ideas. • Agree how the ideas will be elicited – in a round, or by shouting out, or writing on Post-Its.
Materials required:	• Flip chart. • Post-Its (optional).

General rules of brainstorming

1 Clearly state the purpose of the activity.
2 Each person takes a turn, expressing one idea at a time.
3 No-one to criticise or comment.
4 Every idea is accepted as a good one.
5 It is all right to pass if you have nothing to say.
6 Record all ideas verbatim, in a visible place to stimulate new ideas in the group. Do not paraphrase or reword.
7 Seek clarification of an idea where it would help the group.
8 Group together similar concepts if appropriate.

Variations

Free-form brainstorming: anyone can offer an idea as soon as it comes to mind. This produces a relaxed atmosphere and encourages creativity, although not all may contribute. It may be difficult to write quickly enough to keep up with the flow of ideas. Consider enlisting a scribe, or even two, to help out.

Structured brainstorming: ideas are solicited in a round (p. 79) with each member speaking in turn. This is more rigid in format and may inhibit spontaneity.

Silent brainstorming: ideas are written on Post-Its – one idea per Post-It – and then displayed for all to see. All have an equal 'voice'. Some more reticent members might feel more confident about contributing but group synergy is lost. The Post-Its can be grouped in a variety of ways and the volume and spread can be a graphic illustration of the nature or scope of a problem.

The product of brainstorming is a list of ideas which can then be discussed.

Technique:	**A round**
Purpose:	• To gain the views of the whole group, in a systematic way, with all views being accorded equal status. • May be useful for information gathering, eliciting responses to an idea or activity, or sharing feelings about a proposed development. • Can also be used as an ice breaker, where each member of the group is asked a simple question so that they make their first contribution of the meeting in a relatively non-threatening atmosphere.
Tips for use:	• Consider how long this activity will take and ensure that momentum can be sustained throughout. • You may have to limit contributions if the group is large (more than 10 people) by suggesting that everyone talks for no more than one minute or gives one idea only. • All members should be encouraged to say something in the first round, even if it is to express their agreement or disagreement with points previously raised. • If the group would benefit, it may be useful to keep going round the group until all ideas are exhausted. • You, a Facilitator colleague, or a volunteer can record all contributions on a flip chart.
Materials required:	• Flip chart.

The Facilitator poses the question and asks that each member of the group, in turn, replies. All ideas are to be accepted without comment at this stage, the activity ending either once all ideas are exhausted or a time limit has been reached. The question might be, 'What is good about our practice meetings?'

Chapter 6

Qualities, skills and opportunities

Summary

In this chapter we bring together many of the ideas already discussed, and summarise the key messages of the book.

Sections of this chapter highlight:

- the essential qualities of a Facilitator
- opportunities to facilitate within your own practice
- maximising the benefit of working in groups
- the skills of reflection and feedback.

If you have read through the pack chronologically, this chapter should help to establish the main points in your mind or stimulate you to revisit certain chapters.

Please bear in mind that becoming more facilitative or acting effectively in the formal Facilitator role requires skills which need time and practice to develop. Personal qualities and individual style play a significant part and no two Facilitators operate in exactly the same way.

The aim in this handbook has been to heighten awareness of the types of behaviour and the specific interventions which underpin facilitation, and to suggest some areas of practice life where facilitation might be appropriate or necessary. A range of tools have been included to help progress working more effectively in groups.

The essential qualities of a Facilitator

In different settings, and in a variety of ways, Facilitators help groups function more effectively. A useful way to describe their work is:

'Facilitation is the provision of opportunity, resources, encouragement and support for the group to succeed in achieving its own objectives and to do this through enabling the group to take control and responsibility for the way they proceed.'

(Bentley, 1994)

In the NHS, Facilitators have helped groups by offering a wide range of practical assistance and moral support. They have provided ideas, information, advice, direction, resources, support, training and tools and worked with practices in areas of both clinical and organisational development.

Facilitators' skills are rooted in a desire and commitment to work for the benefit of the particular group or organisation and in an understanding of how the effectiveness of group processes can be maximised by paying attention to certain key aspects of:

- planning
- making sense of what is going on
- structuring activities
- dealing with difficult issues
- promoting the well being of the group
- recognising the achievements of the group.

The predominant skills and qualities are typically described as being:

- flexibility of style
- respect for the autonomy of others
- honesty and reliability
- neutrality and objectivity
- sensitivity to others and empathy
- caring, warmth and genuineness in approach
- knowledge of the context and group processes
- ability to provide orientation in the course of work
- enthusiasm and positive attitude to the job in hand
- in possession of a repertoire of techniques and tools for interpersonal and group development
- skill in dealing with conflict.

Regardless of title, *anyone* working in a group can demonstrate, and make deliberate use of, such skills and qualities for the benefit of that group.

Opportunities to facilitate within your own practice

When working in groups in your own practice you may be given the opportunity to take on the formal role of Facilitator. This will entail acting in a slightly different way from normal and the exact role should be made explicit to others so that there is no confusion. For example, you may facilitate a review of practice meetings to assess and improve on their effectiveness. You might also formally set up a new group, working with that group to establish its mode of operation. Or you may take on the task of organising and facilitating a practice away day. Whatever the situation, your role will be to attend to those practical tasks which create a suitable environment in which to work together – the room layout, the timing, the refreshments, the necessary documents etc – and to provide structure, orientation, tools, training, support, resources, interventions and motivation, as necessary, to maximise the benefits of working in that group.

When acting in this formal role you need to be able to work with, and for, the group without either dominating it or being dominated by it, without imposing your own personal agenda or following your own needs.

One area where many primary healthcare teams or practice groups need facilitation is the *process* of working together. Time and other pressures tend to result in a strong focus on the *task* element – meeting deadlines for action, producing documents like development plans and organising new clinics. Scant attention is paid to issues such as:

* the preferred way of working together
* the goals of the group
* full participation by all group members
* dealing with differences in opinion
* ensuring that agreement is real and not superficial
* reviewing the operation of the group.

The use of *facilitative interventions* will probably be the aspect of the facilitator role least familiar to you. These interventions – deliberate verbal and, sometimes, non-verbal responses to a group situation – can help the group to:

* set the climate
* manage time
* ensure active participation
* maintain energy and alertness
* create the future
* draw out issues

- keep to the task
- deal with unhelpful behaviour
- articulate what is not being said
- identify agreement and disagreement
- encourage learning in the group
- give and receive feedback
- complete an activity.

If you are not in the formal Facilitator role, you can nevertheless be a more facilitative group member by understanding the nature of working in groups, behaving in ways which will help the group to function more effectively and suggesting the use of appropriate tools for the group to use to improve its way of working.

Maximising the benefit of working in groups

Groups have the potential to maximise the benefits of working together if they pay attention to the *process* of working together as well as focusing on the *task* in hand. Certain types of behaviour will help get the job done – proposing strategies for action, seeking others' opinions, summarising discussion, clarifying issues. Other actions help the group work together well – encouraging others, being friendly, admitting your own mistakes, helping others to express their feelings.

It helps to understand that groups go through a process of development from the early days where individuals are unsure or reticent, through a stormy time where there may be conflicting priorities or preferences until the goals become clearer and relationships are established, and then to a fruitful period, where members trust each other and work together well. Discussing and clarifying goals, roles, procedures and relationships help ease the group into productivity.

Where a group has the following attributes:

- a clear purpose
- a commitment by all to that purpose
- a common and inspirational vision
- explicit values
- clear roles and commitments
- active work to be done
- a group identity
- an ability to handle conflict
- a recognition of its own worth,

then great things are possible – the skills, knowledge and experience of all members can be tapped and the group can work together productively and harmoniously. Time is well spent in establishing the task and process of a new group or reviewing the operation of an existing group.

Reflection and feedback

We conclude by encouraging you to think about two further facets of the Facilitator role – those of reflection and feedback.

Experience in the Facilitator role and practice of facilitation skills do not necessarily transform a person into a skilful practitioner. However, being able to reflect on performance and events honestly and with insight, and learning from that process of reflection, help to effect the transition.

As a simple framework for reflection we suggest the following process, based on Gibbs (1988):

A process for reflection

1 Description   *What happened?*

Recall the experience as soon after the event as possible, and write down a description of what happened.

2 Feelings   *What were you thinking and feeling?*

- How aware of the experience were you?
- What were you thinking?
- What assumptions did you make and how valid were they?
- What were you feeling?
- What were your own attitudes and feelings in this situation?
- What aspects of your own behaviour were you aware of?

3 Evaluation   *What was good and bad about the experience?*

- What is your interpretation of this situation at present? 'A waste of time', 'being used', 'not being up to the mark', 'a job well done'?
- Include justifications for your interpretations, for example what factors/knowledge are influencing your judgement?
- Did you recognise these as forming a pattern or echoing previous experience?

Cont

4 Analysis *What sense can you make of the situation?*

We sometimes criticise others to take attention away from our own perceived inadequacies; therefore watch any tendency to make judgements either about others or yourself. Re-evaluate the experience by comparing what you already know and feel about this situation, with other possible related causes. For instance, rather than concentrating on the negative/obstructive feelings and events, focus on the positive aspect of the situation.

5 Conclusion *What else could you have done?*

- How do I now feel about this experience?
- How could I have dealt better with this situation?
- What would have been the consequences of these other choices?

6 Action plan *If it arose again what would you do?*

- What have I learned from the experience?
- How would I ensure my practice was going to change for the better, given a similar situation?

Giving feedback

The role of the Facilitator is often to observe or diagnose and then give feedback. This may be to colleagues with whom you work on a daily basis. Giving feedback sensitively can help a group recognise its shortcomings and identify opportunities and scope for improvement, and encourage a desire to work together more productively.

The final tool is a guide to one method of giving feedback.

Technique:	**Giving feedback**
Purpose:	• To enhance learning in an individual or group.
	• To help others evaluate a course of action or a decision.
	• To enhance self-awareness.
Tips for use:	• Give formal feedback only as part of a procedure or programme agreed with the group.
	• Most people respond to praise, encouragement and recognition.
	• If you preface negative feedback with a positive statement it is usually received more favourably.
	• Feedback should be directed only at things the group or individual can do something about.
	• Detailed feedback gives more opportunity for learning than broad, general statements.
	• Allow the other person to accept or reject your feedback – you cannot impose your beliefs or opinions on others.
	• Offer suggestions for improving on more negative areas.
	• Ask for the group's/individual's ideas on how they might effect change.
	• Take responsibility for feedback that you give – say 'I think' or 'in my opinion'.

A useful format to follow when giving feedback is as follows:

1 Facilitator and group/individual recap on what took place.
2 Together they clarify any matters of fact.
3 The group/individual describes what went well.
4 The Facilitator discusses what was achieved.
5 The group/individual discusses which tasks were not achieved and makes recommendations as to how they might have been achieved.
6 The Facilitator discusses which tasks were not achieved and makes recommendations as to how they might have been achieved.
7 Any differences of opinion are discussed and, if possible, resolved.
8 The group/individual is left with a clear knowledge of strengths and of specific changes which might lead to improvement.

In summary, a Facilitator can help a group to achieve its goals, manage periods of change and work together more harmoniously by guiding the process and by actively nurturing the conditions in which the group will flourish. These facilitation skills are acquired through study, practice and reflection, and this handbook should prove a valuable introduction to that process.

References

Bentley T (1994) *Facilitation: providing opportunities for learning.* McGraw Hill, London.

Bray T (1995) *30 Training Sessions for Effective Meetings.* Gower Publishing, Aldershot.

Duffy M, Griffin E and Bain J (1998) *Facilitating Education and Development: The FED Project. Final Report.* Tayside Centre for General Practice, University of Dundee.

Duffy M and Griffin E (1998) *Facilitation Skills Training Workshop.* Tayside Centre for General Practice, University of Dundee.

Gibbs G (1988) *Learning By Doing: a guide to teaching and learning methods.* Further Education Unit, Oxford Polytechnic.

Grant J, Napier A, Stephen S *et al.* (1998) Integrating audit into primary care: a Tayside initiative. *Health Bulletin.* **56**(5): 822–7.

Hart L (1992) *The Faultless Facilitator.* Kogan Page, London.

Havelock P (1997) Using a facilitator. In: D Pendleton and J Hasler (eds) *Professional Development in General Practice.* Oxford University Press, Oxford.

Heron J (1989) *The Facilitator's Handbook.* Kogan Page, London.

Hooker J (1994) Facilitating primary health care. *Journal of Advanced Nursing.* **19**: 1–3.

Hunter D, Bailey A and Taylor B (1996) *The Facilitation of Groups.* Gower Publishing, Aldershot.

Johnson D and Johnson F (1991) *Joining Together: group theory and group skills.* Prentice-Hall, New Jersey.

McCowan C, Neville RG, Crombie IK *et al.* (1997) The facilitator effect: results from a four year follow-up of children with asthma. *British Journal of General Practice.* **47**: 156–60.

Nilson C (1993) *Team Games for Trainers.* McGraw Hill, New York.

Porritt L (1990) *Interaction Strategies: an introduction for health professionals.* Churchill Livingstone, Edinburgh.

The National Primary Care Facilitation Programme (1998) *Primary Care Facilitation: what is it and what is the evidence of its effectiveness?* NPCFP, Oxford.

RCGP (1998) *The Primary Healthcare Team. Information Sheet No 21.* RCGP, London.

Tayside Audit Resource for Primary Care (1999) *Integrating Audit Programme.* Tayside Primary Care Trust, Dundee.

Woodcock M (1989) *The Team Development Manual.* Gower Publishing, Aldershot.